OXFORD NEUROLOGY LIBRARY

Epilepsy

O N L

OXFORD NEUROLOGY LIBRARY

Epilepsy

by

Simon Shorvon

Professor of Neurology
UCL Institute of Neurology
University College London
Consultant Neurologist
National Hospital for Neurology and Neurosurgery
London, UK

OXFORD
UNIVERSITY PRESS

OXFORD

UNIVERSITY PRESS

Great Clarendon Street, Oxford OX2 6DP

Oxford University Press is a department of the University of Oxford.
It furthers the University's objective of excellence in research, scholarship,
and education by publishing worldwide in

Oxford New York

Auckland Cape Town Dar es Salaam Hong Kong Karachi
Kuala Lumpur Madrid Melbourne Mexico City Nairobi
New Delhi Shanghai Taipei Toronto

With offices in

Argentina Austria Brazil Chile Czech Republic France Greece
Guatemala Hungary Italy Japan Poland Portugal Singapore
South Korea Switzerland Thailand Turkey Ukraine Vietnam

Oxford is a registered trade mark of Oxford University Press
in the UK and in certain other countries

Published in the United States
by Oxford University Press Inc., New York

© Oxford University Press, 2009

British Library Cataloguing in Publication Data

Data available

Library of Congress Cataloging in Publication Data

Data available

Typeset by Newgen Imaging Systems (P) Ltd., Chennai, India
Printed in Great Britain
on acid-free paper by
Ashford Colour Press Ltd., Gosport, Hampshire

ISBN 978-0-19-956004-2

10 9 8 7 6 5 4 3 2

Contents

Preface

Epilepsy is a common and important neurological condition. It affects children and adults and occurs in every major population of the world. Epilepsy is a heterogeneous condition, manifesting on its own or as a complication of other neurological or systemic disease, and its clinical form, severity and outcome vary widely. Treatment has improved considerably in recent years, and the choice of medical therapy has widened greatly. Choice brings complexity, and skill and experience are necessary to make the most of the greater range of treatment options. The purpose of this small volume is to provide a short but comprehensive survey of epilepsy and its management for the busy clinician. It is very definitely intended to be a clinical tool—and what is provided is clinical information rather than data relevant to research or experimental study. I have tried to provide as much factual information as possible, in a digestible form, and to avoid longwinded or complex description. Such parsimony has drawbacks—of simplification and generalization particularly—but aids clinical utility. Diagnosis, treatment and counselling are especially emphasized, for it is in these areas that accurate data and clinical skill are particularly needed. I have tried to tabulate information where possible, particularly in the field of therapeutics and pharmacokinetics, to aid rapid reference. The book, it is to be hoped, will be useful for generalists, specialists and trainees—in the many clinical settings in which patients with epilepsy appear.

Please note that many of the drug doses recommended are different (usually lower) than those in the regulatory formularies or the manufacturer's literature. This is because, after licensing, experience in clinical practice frequently leads to different dosage regimens than those initially licensed. What I have attempted to give here is a reflection of current UK specialist practice, as far as this is possible. In emergency therapy particularly, unlicensed usage of drugs is often widespread—and this too is reflected in this book. Where possible I have pointed out where a particular indication or regimen is unlicensed. Some information, especially in relation to pharmaceutical products (for instance, the form of product preparations), varies from country to country and international data is provided where feasible. The information in the book has been checked as far as is possible, but please note that errors may have been inadvertently overlooked (for instance in pharmacological, pharmacokinetic or therapeutic data) and the reader is advised to refer to the published information from the manufacturers, reference works and regulatory agencies. Some of the data is taken from other works (Shorvon SD. *Handbook of Epilepsy treatment* (2nd ed). Blackwell Science, Oxford

2005; Shorvon SD, Perucca E, Engel J. *The treatment of Epilepsy*. (3rd ed) Wiley-Blackwell, Oxford 2009; Clarke C, Howard R, Rossor M, Shorvon SD. *Neurology: a Queen Square Textbook*. Wiley-Blackwell. 2009) and I am heavily indebted to these larger works. I would also like to thank Peter Stevenson and Dominic Stow at Oxford University Press for their work on this book, and also Dr Carol A. Candlish for her careful checking of the therapeutic data. As ever, final thanks too must go to my colleagues and patients, for writing a text such as this would be meaningless or impossible without the experience gained from a long-standing and large clinical practice.

Simon Shorvon, London 2009

Abbreviations

ACTH	adrenocorticotropic hormone
AVM	aerteriovenous malformation
CNS	central nervous system
CSAG	Clinical Standards Advisory Group
CSF	cerebrospinal fluid
CT	computer tomography
DBS	deep brain stimulation
DVLA	Driving and Vehicle Licensing Agency
ECG	electrocardiogram
EEG	electroencephalogram
EPC	epilepsia partialis continua
FLAIR	fluid attenuated inversion recovery
GABA	gamma-aminobutyric acid
GTCS	generalized tonic-clonic seizure
HIV	human immunodeficiency virus
IGE	Idiopathic Generalized Epilepsy
IgG	immunoglobulin
ILAE	International League Against Epilepsy
IM	intramuscular
IQ	intelligence quotient
ITU	intensive treatment unit
IV	intravenous
JME	juvenile myoclonic epilepsy
LSD	lysergic acid diethylamide
LVA	low-voltage activated
NMDA	N-methyl D-aspartate
MDME	methyllenedioxy-methamphetamine
MHD	monohydroxy derivative metabolite
MRC	Medical Research Council
MRI	magnetic resonance imaging
NCC	neurocysticercosis

NEAD	non-epileptic attack disorder
PME	progressive myoclonic epilepsy
PET	positron emission tomography
REM	rapid eye movement
SLE	systemic lupus erythematosus
SPECT	single photon emission computed tomography
SUDEP	sudden unexpected death in epilepsy
TLE	temporal lobe epilepsy
VIQ	verbal intelligence quotient

Chapter 1

Definition and frequency of epilepsy

Key points

- Epilepsy is one of the most common neurological conditions. In a typical Western population of 1 million people, there will be 5,000 people with epilepsy and 500 new cases each year.
- Epilepsy can take many forms and has many causes.
- The highest incidence rates are in children and in the elderly. It also occurs with a high frequency in people with learning disability.
- Although the prognosis is generally good, the mortality rate in epilepsy is higher than in the general population. *Sudden unexpected death in epilepsy* (SUDEP) is a particular problem occurring in patients prone to tonic-clonic seizures, at a frequency of approximately 1 case per 2,500 persons per year in mild epilepsy to 1 case per 100 persons per year in severe epilepsy.

1.1 Definitions

1.1.1 Epileptic seizure (epileptic fit)

An epileptic seizure is defined as *the transient clinical manifestation that results from an episode of epileptic neuronal activity*. The epileptic neuronal activity is a specific dysfunction, characterized by abnormal synchronization, excessive excitation, and/or inadequate inhibition, and can affect small or large neuronal populations (aggregates). The nature of the clinical manifestations depends on the part of the brain involved in the epileptic neuronal discharge, and the physiology and spread of the discharge.

1.1.2 Epilepsy

Epilepsy is defined as a *disorder of brain characterized by an ongoing liability to recurrent epileptic seizures*. For pragmatic reasons, for the purposes of epidemiological research and in a clinical setting, patients with single seizures, provoked seizures, or febrile seizures are usually excluded. Active epilepsy is defined as epilepsy in which a seizure has occurred in the previous 2 years.

1.1.3 **Provoked seizure**

A provoked seizure (synonym: acute symptomatic seizures) is defined as a seizure which has an obvious and immediate preceding cause (for instance, an acute systemic or metabolic disturbance, or exposure to toxins or drugs) or which is the direct result of a recent acute cerebral damage (for instance, stroke, trauma, infection).

1.1.4 **Febrile seizure**

A febrile seizure is an epileptic event that occurs in the context of an acute rise in body temperature, usually in children between 6 months and 6yrs of age, in whom there is no evidence of intracranial infection or other defined intracranial cause.

1.1.5 **Epileptic encephalopathy**

This is defined as a clinical state in which the changes in cognition or other cerebral function are, at least in part, likely to be directly due to ongoing epileptic processes in the brain. The epileptic encephalopathies are commoner in children than in adults.

1.1.6 **Idiopathic, symptomatic, and cryptogenic epilepsy**

Epilepsy can have many causes. Where the cause is clearly identified, the epilepsy is categorized as *symptomatic* (i.e. of known cause). Where no cause is known, the epilepsy is known as *cryptogenic* (i.e. hidden cause). Where the epilepsy is predominately of genetic (or presumed genetic) origin, it is categorized as *idiopathic*.

1.1.7 **Status epilepticus**

This is defined as a condition in which epileptic seizures continue, or are repeated without recovery, for a period of 30min or more. There has been recent debate about what is the minimum duration of seizures necessary to define this condition, with suggestions ranging from 5min to 60min, but 30min is the usual current formulation. Status epilepticus can take many forms, both convulsive and nonconvulsive. Tonic-clonic status epilepticus (convulsive status epilepticus) should be treated as a medical emergency and carries a mortality rate of approximately 20%. Approximately 60% of cases of tonic-clonic status occur *de novo*, in persons without a history of epilepsy who sustain a sudden, severe brain insult, and the outcome and clinical features are to a large extent, in these cases, dependent on the underlying cause.

1.2 **Epidemiology of epilepsy**

1.2.1 **Frequency of epilepsy**

Epilepsy is a common condition. The incidence of epilepsy has been found to be in the region of 50–80 cases per 100,000 persons per year in most studies. The point prevalence is approximately 4–10 cases per 1,000 persons. Epilepsy is more common in underdeveloped countries, perhaps because of poorer perinatal care and standards of nutrition and public hygiene, and the greater risk of brain injury, cerebral infection, or other acquired cerebral conditions. The frequency of epilepsy is also slightly higher in lower socio-economic classes, and may be slightly more likely in males compared to females. However, epilepsy has been found in all parts of the world and can affect all strata in a population. The similarities of the condition in most populations are more striking than any differences.

The incidence of seizures is highest in the first year of life. The rates remain high in childhood and then fall to low levels in early adult life. The rates rise again in late life.

1.2.2 **Prognosis**

Approximately 60% of the patients diagnosed as having epilepsy will cease having seizures within 5yrs of diagnosis, and 50% will have withdrawn therapy. In approximately 20% of cases, epilepsy, once developed, never remits. In the other 20%, the course of the condition will be punctuated by periods of remission and relapse. Even in those whose epilepsy does not remit, however, the frequency and severity of seizures can be greatly reduced by therapy.

1.2.3 **Mortality**

The standardized mortality rates are two to three times higher in patients with epilepsy than in the unaffected individuals in the population. The excess mortality is due largely to the underlying cause of the epilepsy (for instance, patients with epilepsy because of a brain tumour have a higher mortality due to the tumour). However, some deaths are directly due to seizures and there are also higher rates of accidents and of suicide.

Sudden unexpected death in epilepsy (SUDEP) is a particular problem. It occurs at a frequency that ranges from one death per 2,500 persons per year in mild epilepsy to one death per 100 patients per year amongst those with severe and intractable epilepsy. It is thought that SUDEP usually occurs in the aftermath of a major convulsion and is due to either a cardiac arrhythmia or a central respiratory arrest because of the seizure. It is more common in young adults with epilepsy, in those having seizures whilst asleep and unaccompanied, in those with frequent or severe convulsive seizures, in those with learning disability or symptomatic epilepsy.

1.2.4 **Epilepsy and learning disability**

Approximately one-third to one half of children, and approximately one-fifth of adults, with epilepsy have additional learning disability. Epilepsy occurs in approximately 20% of those with learning disability: 7%–18% of those with intelligence quotients (IQs) rated between 50 and 70, and 35%–44% in those with IQ ratings below 50. Eighteen percentage of adults with newly diagnosed epilepsy show additional dementia and 6% motor disabilities (usually hemiplegia due to stroke) and 6% severe psychiatric disorders. Approximately one in fifteen persons with epilepsy is dependent on others for daily living because of epilepsy or the associated handicaps.

1.2.5 The features of epilepsy in a general population

An approximate breakdown of numerical aspects of epilepsy in a typical western population of 1,000,000 persons is shown in Table 1.1. Approximately two thirds of cases have seizures less than once a month and require only minor medical input. Approximately 50% of cases have had no seizures in the prior 12 months. Approximately 5%–10% of patients have seizures at a greater than weekly frequency, require intensive medical resources for their epilepsy, and incur significant medical costs. In terms of direct medical care costs, epilepsy accounts for approximately 0.25% of General Practitioner (GP) costs, 0.63% of hospital costs, and 0.95% of pharmaceutical costs (data from the UK National Health Service). Epilepsy results in social exclusion and isolation, and causes problems in education, employment, personal development, personal relationships and family life, and dependency. These secondary handicaps are to a large extent culturally determined, and are discussed further in Chapter 9.

Table 1.1 Epilepsy in a population of 1,000,000 persons (approximate estimates)	
Incident cases (new cases each year):	
Febrile seizures (annual incidence rate 50/100,000)	500
Single seizures (annual incidence rate 20/100,000)	200
Epilepsy (annual incidence rate 50/100,000)	500
Prevalent cases (cases with established epilepsy):	
Active epilepsy (prevalence rate 5/1,000)	5,000
Epilepsy in remission	15,000
Severity of epilepsy (in active epilepsy):	
More than one seizure a week	15%
Between one seizure a week and one a month	25%
Less than one seizure a month	60%
Type of seizures:	
Partial seizures alone	15%
Partial and secondarily generalized	60%
Generalized tonic-clonic	20%
Other generalized seizures	5%
Medical care required (in prevalent cases):	
Occasional medical attention	65%
Regular medical attention	30%
Residential or institutional care	5%

References and further reading

Annegers JF, Hauser WA, and Elveback LR (1979). Remission of seizures and relapse in patients with epilepsy. *Epilepsia*, **30**, 729–37.

Annegers JF, Hauser WA, Lee JR, and Rocca WA (1995). Secular trends and birth cohort effects in unprovoked seizures in Rochester, Minnesota: 1935–1984. *Epilepsia*, **36**, 575–9.

Anonymous (1981). Proposal for revised clinical and electroencephalographic classification of epileptic seizures. From the Commission on Classification and Terminology of the International League Against Epilepsy. *Epilepsia*, **22**(4), 489–501.

Anonymous (1989). Proposal for revised classification of epilepsies and epileptic syndromes. Commission on Classification and Terminology of the International League Against Epilepsy. *Epilepsia*, **30**(4), 389–99.

Clinical Standards Advisory Group (CSAG) (2000). Standards of care for patients with epilepsy in the UK. Department of Health.

Cockerell OC, Johnson AJ, Goodridge DMG, Sander JWAS, and Shorvon SD (1997). Prognosis of epilepsy: a review and further analysis of the first nine years of the British National General Practice Study of Epilepsy, a prospective population-based study. *Epilepsia*, **38**, 31–46.

Eriksson KJ and Koivikko MJ (1997). Prevalence, classification, and severity of epilepsy and epileptic syndromes in children. *Epilepsia*, **38**, 1275–82.

Forsgren L, Edvinsson S-O, Blomquist HK, Heijbel J, and Sidenvall R (1990). Epilepsy in a population of mentally retarded children and adults. *Epilepsy Research*, **6**, 234–48.

Forsgren L, Bucht G, Eriksson S, and Bergmark L (1996). Incidence and clinical characterization of unprovoked seizures in adults: a prospective population-based study. *Epilepsia*, **37**, 224–9.

Gaitatzis A, Johnson AL, Chadwick DW, Shorvon SD, and Sander JW (2004). Life expectancy in people with newly diagnosed epilepsy. *Brain*, **127**, 2427–32q.

Hauser WA, Annegers J, and Elveback L (1980). Mortality in patients with epilepsy. *Epilepsia*, **21**, 399–412.

Hauser WA, Annegers JF, and Kurland LT (1991). Prevalence of epilepsy in Rochester, Minnesota: 1940–1980. *Epilepsia*, **32**, 429–45.

Hauser WA, Rich SS, Lee JRJ, Annegers JF, and Anderson VE (1998). Risk of recurrent seizures after two unprovoked seizures. *The New England Journal of Medicine*, **338**, 429–34.

Lhatoo SD, Johnson AL, Goodridge DM, MacDonald BK, Sander JWAS, and Shorvon SD (2001). Mortality in epilepsy in the first 11–14 years after diagnosis: multivariate analysis of a long-term, prospective, population-based cohort. *Annals of Neurology*, **49**, 336–44.

Lindsten H, Stenlund H, and Forsgren L (2001). Remission of seizures in a population-based adult cohort with a newly diagnosed unprovoked epileptic seizure. *Epilepsia*, **42**, 1025–30.

MacDonald BK, Cockerell OC, Sander JWAS, and Shorvon SD (2000). The incidence and lifetime prevalence of neurological disorders in a prospective community-based study in the UK. *Brain*, **123**, 665–76.

Shorvon SD (2005). The clinical forms and causes of epilepsy. In SD Shorvon, ed. *Handbook of epilepsy treatment*, 2nd edn. Blackwell Science, Oxford.

Chapter 2

Clinical forms of epilepsy

Key points

- Epilepsy is usually classified according to (a) seizure type and (b) syndrome, although classification by anatomical focus (in partial epilepsy) and by aetiology is also useful.
- Seizure type is subdivided into partial and generalized forms. Partial epilepsies account for approximately 75% of all cases.
- The commonest syndrome is *Idiopathic Generalized Epilepsy* (IGE) that has highly specific clinical features.
- There are a number of important childhood epilepsy syndromes with specific clinical features, some benign and some very severe.
- Febrile seizures occur in approximately 5% of children and are usually benign. Approximately 2%–7.5% of children develop epilepsy after febrile convulsions.

Epilepsy can present in different ways and can take many different forms. There are two common methods of classification: one of 'seizure type' and the other of 'epilepsy syndrome'. The aetiology of the epilepsy is also important—and this is covered in Chapter 3. When diagnosing a patient, the seizure type and syndrome, and the aetiology should be clearly identified.

2.1 Seizure type

The seizure type classification of the *International League Against Epilepsy* (ILAE) is the most commonly used classification scheme for epilepsy worldwide. In this scheme, seizures are divided into generalized and partial categories (Box 2.1).

Generalized seizures are those that arise from large areas of cortex simultaneously in both hemispheres and have no focal cerebral onset. Consciousness is always lost. They are subdivided into six categories.

Partial seizures are those that arise in specific often small loci of cerebral cortex in one hemisphere (the epileptic focus). They are divided into simple partial seizures, defined by the absence of alteration of consciousness, and complex partial seizures in which consciousness is impaired or lost.

Box 2.1 The 1981 ILAE classification of seizure type

I Partial (focal, local) seizures

A Simple partial seizures:
  1 With motor signs
  2 With somatosensory or special sensory symptoms
  3 With autonomic symptoms or signs
  4 With psychic symptoms

B Complex partial seizures:
  1 Simple partial onset followed by impairment of consciousness
  2 With impairment of consciousness at onset

C Partial seizures evolving to secondarily generalized seizures (tonic-clonic, tonic, or clonic):
  1 Simple partial seizures evolving to generalized seizures
  2 Complex partial seizures evolving to generalized seizures
  3 Simple partial seizures evolving to complex partial seizures evolving to   generalized seizures

II Generalized seizures (convulsive and nonconvulsive)

A Absence seizures:
  1 Typical absence seizures
  2 Atypical absence seizures

B Myoclonic seizures

C Clonic seizures

D Tonic seizures

E Tonic-clonic seizures

F Atonic seizures (Astatic seizures)

III Unclassified epileptic seizures

Seizures also spread and may evolve from one category to another. A secondarily generalized seizure is defined as a generalized seizure (usually tonic-clonic) in which the epileptic discharges start as a focal seizure and then evolve into a generalized attack. Simple partial seizures may spread to become complex partial seizures and can spread to become secondarily generalized. When a simple partial seizure evolves in this way, it forms the 'aura' of the complex partial or secondarily generalized seizure.

2.1.1 **Partial seizures**

2.1.1.1 *Simple partial seizures*

Simple partial seizures are defined as partial seizures in which consciousness is not impaired. They are due to focal cerebral disease

ILAE, International League Against Epilepsy.

and can occur at any age. Any cortical region may be affected, the most common sites being the frontal and temporal lobes. Their clinical form depends on the cerebral location of the seizure discharge and the symptoms are useful in predicting the anatomical localization of the seizures. Any form of pathology can result in the same seizure form. Most simple partial seizures last only a few seconds. The manifestations can include the following:

- (a) Motor manifestations—jerking, spasms, posturing, version, anarthria or dysarthria, respiratory arrest
- (b) Somatosensory or special sensory manifestations (simple hallucinations)—these take the form of tingling or numbness, or less commonly an electrical shock-like feeling, burning, pain, or a feeling of heat (in epilepsy involving central or parietal regions), flashing lights and colours (if the epilepsy involves the calcarine cortex). A rising epigastric sensation is the commonest manifestation of a simple partial seizure arising in the mesial temporal lobe
- (c) Autonomic manifestations—these include changes in skin colour, blood pressure, heart rate, pupil size, and piloerection
- (d) Psychic manifestations—these can take various forms, and occur particularly in epilepsy arising from a temporal foci. There are six principal categories:
  - *Dysphasic symptoms* are prominent if cortical speech areas (frontal or temporoparietal) are affected.
  - *Dysmnestic symptoms* (disturbance of memory): for instance, flashbacks, *déjà vu*, *jamais vu*, or panoramic experiences (recollections of previous experiences, former life, or childhood)
  - *Cognitive symptoms* include dreamy states and sensations of unreality or depersonalization
  - *Affective symptoms* include fear (the commonest affective symptom), depression, anger, and irritability
  - *Illusions* of size (macropsia, micropsia): shape, weight, distance, or sound are usually features of temporal or parieto-occipital epileptic foci.
  - *Structured hallucinations* of visual, auditory, gustatory, or olfactory forms, which can be crude or elaborate, are usually due to epileptic discharges in the temporal or parieto-occipital association areas. Visual hallucinations can vary greatly in sophistication. Auditory hallucinations also vary in complexity, and most commonly occur in seizures arising in Herschel's gyrus.

Todd's paralysis is a term used to refer to a reversible unilateral weakness, lasting minutes or hours, that occurs after a partial seizure, which involves motor cortex.

2.1.1.2 *Complex Partial Seizures*

Complex partial seizures arise from the temporal lobe in approximately 60% of cases, the frontal lobe in approximately 30%, and from other cortical areas in approximately 10% of cases. In one series, the ictal phase lasted between 3 and 343sec (mean of 54sec), the post-ictal phase 3–767sec, and the total seizure duration 5–998sec (mean of 128sec), although longer seizures (sometimes lasting hours) are occasionally encountered.

Complex partial seizures, in their complete form, have three components:

1. **Aura**—these are in effect simple partial seizures. They can take any of the forms described earlier. The aura is usually short-lived, lasting a few seconds or so. Many patients with partial seizures experience both isolated auras (simple partial seizures) and full-blown complex partial seizures.

2. **Altered consciousness**—this is known as 'the absence'. It can follow the aura or occur without an aura. The patient ceases activity (motor arrest) and becomes motionless and inaccessible, and appears vacant or glazed (the 'motionless stare'). The absence in complex partial seizures can be mistaken for a generalized absence (and the term *petit mal* is frequently, wrongly used to cover both) (see Table 2.1).

3. **Automatisms**—these are defined as involuntary motor actions that occur during or in the aftermath of epileptic seizures, in a state of impaired awareness. The patient is totally amnesic for the events of the automatism. Automatisms are most common in temporal and frontal lobe seizures. They are usually subdivided into:

- *Oro-alimentary automatisms*—orofacial movements such as chewing, lip smacking, swallowing, or drooling. These are commonest in partial seizures of mesial temporal origin.
- *Mimicry automatisms*—including displays of laughter or fear, anger or excitement.
- *Gestural and motor automatisms*—fiddling movements with the hands, tapping, patting, or rubbing, ordering and tidying movements. Complex actions such as undressing are also quite common as are genitally directed actions. Motor activity involving the upper limbs is commonest in partial seizures of temporal lobe origin, and involving the legs in partial seizures of frontal lobe origin.
- *Ambulatory automatisms*—walking, circling, running. These are commonest in seizures of frontal lobe origin.
- *Verbal automatisms*—meaningless sounds, humming, whistling, grunting, words which may be repeated, formed sentences.
- *Responsive automatisms*—are quasi-purposeful behaviour, seemingly responsive to environmental stimuli.

Table 2.1 Clinical features that help differentiate typical generalized absence seizures from complex partial seizures

	Generalized absence seizure	Complex partial seizure
Age of onset	Childhood or early adult	Any age
Aetiology/syndrome	Idiopathic Generalized Epilepsy	Any focal aetiology (or cryptogenic epilepsy)
Underlying focal anatomical lesion	None	Often present (usually in temporal or frontal lobe)
Duration of attack	Short (usually <15sec)	Longer, usually several minutes
Other clinical features	Usually slight (blinking, nodding, or mild loss of tone)	Can be prominent; aura and motor automatism
Post-ictal	None	Confusion, headache, emotional disturbance are common
Frequency	May be very numerous (hundreds a day)	Usually less frequent (usually less than several per day) with marked clustering
Ictal and interictal EEG	3Hz spike/wave	Variable focal disturbance
Photosensitivity	10%–30%	None
Effect of hyperventilation on EEG	Often marked increase (especially if off treatment)	None, modest increase

EEG = electroencephalogram.

It is often important to establish the laterality of a complex partial seizure, not least as part of a work-up for surgical treatment. Certain signs are of significant lateralizing value and include ictal dystonic spasm of one hand or arm (contralateral to the side of seizure onset); unilateral upper limb automatism (ipsilateral to the side of seizure onset); post-ictal dysphasia (seizure onset in the dominant hemisphere); ictal speech (seizure onset in the non-dominant hemisphere); post-ictal Todd's paralysis or sensory disturbance (contralateral to the side of seizure onset). Version of the head or eyes is a useful lateralizing sign only if it is at the onset of a seizure, with consciousness preserved, in which situation it indicates a contralateral frontal lobe seizure onset. Most other signs are too inconsistent to be very useful as lateralizing or localizing features.

2.1.2 **Generalized seizures**

There are six categories of generalized seizure. In all, consciousness is impaired from the onset of the attack (owing to the extensive cortical and subcortical involvement), motor changes are bilateral and more or less symmetric, and the EEG patterns are bilateral and grossly synchronous and symmetrical over both hemispheres.

2.1.2.1 *Typical absence seizures (petit mal seizures)*

The seizure comprises an abrupt sudden loss of consciousness (the absence) and cessation of all motor activity. Tone is usually preserved, and there is no fall. The patient is not in contact with the environment, inaccessible, and often appears glazed or vacant. The attack ends as abruptly as it started, and previous activity is resumed as if nothing had happened. There is no confusion, but the patient is often unaware that an attack has occurred. Most absence seizures (>80%) last for less than 10sec. Other clinical phenomena including blinking, slight clonic movements of the trunk or limbs, alterations in tone, and/or brief automatisms can occur particularly in longer attacks. The attacks can be repeated, sometimes hundreds of times a day, often cluster and are often worse when the patient is awakening or drifting off to sleep. Absences may be precipitated by fatigue, drowsiness, relaxation, photic stimulation, or hyperventilation. Typical absence seizures develop in childhood or adolescence and are encountered almost exclusively in the syndrome of IGE.

2.1.2.2 *Atypical absence seizures*

These take the form of loss of awareness (absence) and hypo-motor behaviour. They are longer, with less complete loss of awareness and with more marked associated tone changes or motor activity than in typical absence seizures. The onset and cessation of the attacks are not so abrupt. Amnesia may not be complete and the subject may be partially responsive. The patient appears relatively inaccessible, may be ambulant although often stumbling or clumsy and needing guidance or support, and there can be atonic, clonic, or tonic phenomena, autonomic disturbance, and automatisms. The attacks can wax and wane and may be of long duration. Atypical absences occur in the symptomatic epilepsies, are usually associated with learning disability, other neurological abnormalities, or multiple seizure types. They form part of the Lennox–Gastaut syndrome and they may occur at any age (Table 2.2).

Table 2.2 Clinical features differentiating typical and atypical absence seizures

	Typical absence seizure	Atypical absence seizure
Context	Otherwise no other neurological features	Usually in context of learning difficulty, and other neurological abnormalities
Aetiology	Idiopathic Generalized Epilepsy	Lennox–Gastaut syndrome and other severe secondarily generalized and cryptogenic generalized epilepsies
Consciousness	Totally lost	Often only partially impaired
Focal signs in seizures	Nil	May be present
Onset/offset of seizures	Abrupt	Often gradual
Coexisting seizure types	Sometimes tonic-clonic and myoclonic	Mixed seizure disorder is common with all other seizure types

2.1.3 Myoclonic seizures

A myoclonic seizure is a brief contraction of a muscle, muscle group, or several muscle groups due to a cortical discharge. It can be single or repetitive, varying in severity from an almost imperceptible twitch to a severe jerking resulting, for instance, in a sudden fall or the propulsion of handheld objects (the 'flying saucer' syndrome). Recovery is immediate, and the patient often maintains that consciousness was not lost.

Myoclonic seizures occur in very different types of epilepsy. They are one of the three seizure types in the syndrome of IGE (the other two being absence and tonic-clonic seizures) and in this syndrome, the myoclonus usually has a strong diurnal pattern, occurring mainly in the first few hours after waking or when dropping off to sleep. Myoclonic seizures also occur in the childhood epileptic encephalo-pathies (e.g. Lennox–Gastaut syndrome), in epilepsy associated with other forms of learning disability, focal occipital or frontal epilepsy, and in progressive myoclonic epilepsies.

2.1.4 Clonic seizures

Clonic seizures take the form of clonic jerking which is often asym-metric and irregular. Clonic seizures are most frequent in neonates, infants, or young children, and are always symptomatic.

2.1.5 **Tonic seizures**

Tonic seizures take the form of a tonic muscle contraction with altered consciousness without a clonic phase. The tonic contraction causes extension of the neck, contraction of the facial muscles, upturning of the eyeballs, apnea, spasm of the proximal upper limb muscles causing abduction and elevation of the semi-flexed arms. There may be a cry. Tonic seizures last less than 60sec. Tonic seizures occur at all ages in the setting of diffuse cerebral damage, learning disability, and are invariably associated with other seizure types. They are the characteristic and defining seizure type in the Lennox–Gastaut syndrome.

2.1.6 **Tonic-clonic seizures (grand mal seizures)**

This is the classic form of epileptic convulsion. The seizure is initiated by loss of consciousness, and sometimes the epileptic cry. The patient will fall if standing, there is a brief period of tonic flexion, and then a longer phase of rigidity and axial extension, with the eyes rolled up, the jaw clamped shut, the limbs stiff and extended, and the fists either clenched or held in the *main d'accoucheur* position. Respiration ceases and cyanosis is common. This tonic stage lasts on average 10–30sec and is followed by the clonic phase, during which convulsive movements usually of all four limbs, jaw, and facial muscles occur; breathing can be stertorous; and saliva (sometimes blood stained owing to tongue-biting) may froth from the mouth. The convulsive movements decrease in frequency (eventually to about four clonic jerks per second), and increase in amplitude as the attack progresses. Autonomic features such as flushing, changes in blood pressure, changes in pulse rate, and increased salivation are common. The clonic phase lasts between 30sec and 60sec and is followed by a further brief tonic contraction of all muscles, sometimes with incontinence. The final phase lasts between 2min and 30min and is characterized by flaccidity of the muscles. Consciousness is slowly regained. The plantar responses are usually extensor at this time and the tendon jerks are diminished. Confusion is invariable in the post-ictal phase. The patient often has a severe headache, feels dazed and extremely unwell, and often lapses into deep sleep. On awakening minutes or hours later, there may be no residual symptoms or, more commonly, persisting headache, dysthymia, lethargy, muscle aching, soreness and stiffness of limbs and jaw.

Tonic-clonic seizures can result in injury. The tongue-biting is typically on the lateral aspect of the tongue. A posterior dislocation of the shoulder can occur and is said to be diagnostic of a seizure.

Tonic-clonic seizures can occur at any age and are encountered in many different types of epilepsy, including IGE, symptomatic generalized epilepsies, epileptic encephalopathies, in various epilepsy syndromes, in febrile convulsions, and in acute symptomatic seizures. They have no pathological specificity.

2.1.7 **Atonic seizures**

The most severe form is the classic drop attack (astatic seizure) in which all postural tone is suddenly lost causing collapse to the ground like a rag doll. The tone change can be more restricted, resulting, for instance, in nodding of the head, a bowing movement, or sagging at the knee. The seizures are short and are followed by immediate recovery. Longer (inhibitory) atonic attacks can develop in a stepwise fashion with progressively increasing nodding, sagging, or folding. The seizures occur at any age, and are always associated with diffuse cerebral damage, learning disability, and are common in severe symptomatic epilepsies (especially in the Lennox–Gastaut syndrome and in myoclonic astatic epilepsy).

2.2 **Anatomical location of partial seizures**

The forms of partial seizures vary according to their anatomical location. This is important when considering surgical therapy, although not for medical treatment as the indications for antiepileptic drugs are the same whatever the seizure location. Clinical localization is often difficult, and not as precise as often postulated, because of the tendency of epileptic seizures to spread widely and so involve many areas of the brain, and also because many partial seizures are underpinned by a widely distributed abnormal neuronal network rather than a single focus of epileptic tissue.

2.2.1 **Temporal lobe**

The temporal lobe is the commonest site for partial seizures. Differentiation of mesial and lateral temporal lobe epilepsy is important for surgical therapy, but the features overlap considerably and a clear distinction is often impossible. The commonest seizure type is the mesial temporal seizure (Box 2.2).

2.2.2 **Frontal lobe**

Partial seizures of frontal lobe origin have a number of characteristic features which differentiate these from temporal lobe epilepsy (Box 2.3) but the features overlap (due to spread) and clinical localization can be unreliable.

Box 2.2 Complex partial seizures of mesial temporal lobe origin

- Tripartite seizure pattern (aura, absence, automatism) in some patients
- Partial awareness commonly preserved, especially in early stages, and slow evolution of seizure
- Auras include visceral, cephalic, gustatory, dysmnestic, affective, perceptual, or autonomic auras
- Dystonic posturing of the contralateral upper limb and ipsilateral automatisms common
- In seizures arising in the dominant temporal lobe, speech arrest during the seizures and dysphasia post-ictally
- Seizures typically last >2min, with a slow evolution and gradual onset/offset
- Autonomic changes (e.g. pallor, redness, and tachycardia) common
- Automatisms are often oro-alimentary or upper limb gestural in form and are sometimes prolonged.
- Post-ictal confusion common
- Seizures tend to cluster
- Secondary generalization (to a tonic-clonic seizure) infrequent
- In patients with hippocampal sclerosis:
    - Past history of febrile convulsions
    - Onset in mid childhood or adolescence
    - Initial response to therapy, lost after several years

Box 2.3 Clinical features of complex partial seizures of frontal lobe origin that help differentiation from complex partial seizures of temporal lobe origin

- Frequent attacks with clustering
- Often nocturnal
- Brief stereotyped seizures (<30sec) with sudden onset and cessation, with rapid evolution and awareness lost at onset
- Absence of complex aura
- Version of head or eye and prominent motor activity
- Prominent complex bilateral motor automatisms involving lower limbs
- Absence of post-ictal confusion
- Frequent secondary generalization
- History of status epilepticus

2.2.3 **Central, parietal, and occipital lobe**

Seizures arise less commonly from these sites, but the features are often characteristic. The seizures arising in the central (peri-rolandic) region have prominent motor features often without loss of consciousness (Box 2.4). Parietal and occipital seizures have specific features when localized to the primary cortices, but overlap with each other and with temporal lobe seizures when localized to the association cortices—an important point as the areas of cortex around the temporo-parieto-occipital boundaries are common sites for seizures (Boxes 2.5 and 2.6).

Box 2.4 **Features of central cortical seizures**

Partial seizures of central origin

- Contralateral clonic jerking (which may or may not march) or spasm
- Posturing, which is often bilateral, and version of head and eyes
- Speech arrest and involvement of bulbar musculature (producing anarthria or choking, gurgling sounds)
- Contralateral sensory symptoms
- Short frequently recurring attacks that cluster, or prolonged seizures with slow progression, and episodes of epilepsia partialis continua
- Post-ictal Todd's paralysis

Box 2.5 **Features of parietal lobe seizures**

- Contralateral somatosensory symptoms (e.g. tingling, numbness, or more complex sensations) which may or may not 'march' (spread through the body)
- Complex illusions and perceptual change
- Auditory changes, distortions, illusions and hallucinations
- Illusions of change in body size/shape, vertigo, feeling of being unable to move
- Visual changes, illusions and hallucinations (e.g. objects, scenes, autoscopia, often moving)

Box 2.6 Features of occipital lobe seizures

- Elementary visual hallucinations in the contralateral visual field. These take the form of flashes, colours, shapes, or patterns. These can grow rapidly in size and extent as the seizure develops.
- Forced head turning usually contralaterally, sometimes accompanied by a sensation of following or looking at a visual hallucination.
- Perceptual change, for instance, of size (micropsia, macropsia), shape, or position
- Loss or dulling of vision (amaurosis)
- Eyelid fluttering, blinking, nystagmus

2.3 **Epilepsy syndromes**

An epileptic syndrome is defined as an epileptic disorder characterized by a cluster of signs and symptoms customarily occurring together. They represent clusters of clinical importance but there is often a complex relationship to underlying aetiology or pathophysiology. Whilst some syndromes represent a single disease, others can have many underlying causes (for instance, the Lennox–Gastaut syndrome); furthermore, the same underlying disease can manifest as different epileptic syndromes (for instance, in tuberose sclerosis). The syndromes are age specific, and over time in individual patients, one epileptic syndrome can evolve into another. Similarly, the same seizure type can occur in very different syndromes (e.g. myoclonic seizures in the benign syndrome of *Juvenile Myoclonic Epilepsy (JME)* and the severe refractory Progressive Myoclonic Epilepsies).

The outline structure of the ILAE classification of the epilepsies and epileptic syndromes is shown in Box 2.7. Within each of these categories a number of epilepsy syndromes are included. A detailed description of all of these is beyond the scope of this small volume. Here several of the most common or the most important are briefly described.

Box 2.7 **ILAE classification of epilepsy syndromes**

1. **Localization-related epilepsies**
   - Idiopathic
   - Symptomatic
   - Cryptogenic
2. **Generalized epilepsies**
   - Idiopathic
   - Symptomatic
   - Cryptogenic
3. **Epilepsies and syndromes undetermined with focal or generalized**
   - Idiopathic
   - Symptomatic
   - Cryptogenic
   - Special syndromes
4. **Situation-related seizures**

2.3.1 Idiopathic Generalized Epilepsy (IGE) (Box 2.8)

The term IGE (synonym: *Primary Generalized Epilepsy*) is used to denote a very common and important group of conditions. These have a characteristic clinical and electrographic pattern and a probable genetic basis. Patients with IGE account for approximately 10%–30% of all those with epilepsy.

The syndrome can be subdivided into different subgroups, although the validity of doing so is open to question. Core clinical features are features shared to a greater or lesser extent by these subgroups (at least those with onset in later childhood or early adult life) and are shown in Box 2.8.

2.3.1.1 Childhood absence epilepsy (synonym: pyknolepsy) is a subgroup which accounts for between 1% and 3% of newly diagnosed epilepsies and up to 10% of childhood epilepsies. In this condition, absence seizures are the predominant seizure type. These start in the early and middle years of childhood (peak age 6–7yrs). The seizures are very brief lasting usually 5–15sec, and in some cases pass unrecognized for long periods. Many can occur in a day, and the seizures tend to cluster. The classical ictal EEG pattern is monotonous, generalized 3Hz spike-wave. Approximately one-third of patients also develop tonic-clonic seizures (GTCS) at a later time. The prognosis is good, and rapid remission on therapy is expected in 80% or more of patients. When followed-up after age 18yrs, only approximately 20% of previously diagnosed patients are still having seizures.

ILAE = International League Against Epilepsy.

> ## Box 2.8 Clinical features of Idiopathic Generalized Epilepsy (IGE)
>
> - 10%–30% of all epilepsy
> - Onset usually in childhood or early adult life
> - Positive family history in some cases
> - Generalized seizure types—myoclonus, generalized absence (*petit mal*), and generalized tonic-clonic seizures
> - Normal EEG background, with intermittent paroxysms of generalized spike-wave or polyspike-wave discharges
> - Ictal EEG shows generalized EEG discharges, either 3Hz spike and wave or polyspike burst
> - Photosensitivity present in some cases (age related)
> - Seizures especially on awakening and during sleep
> - Normal intellect
> - Absence of identifiable underlying structural aetiology
> - Excellent response to therapy (especially to valproate)

2.3.1.2 *Juvenile myoclonic epilepsy*

Juvenile myoclonic epilepsy (synonyms include impulsive *petit mal*; Janz syndrome) is the most common subtype of IGE, and accounts for up to 10% of all epilepsies. The characteristic seizures are brief myoclonic jerks, occurring in the first hour or so after awakening, and usually in bursts. In 80% of cases, the myoclonus develops between the ages of 12yrs and 18yrs (and always between 6yrs and 25yrs, but may be unrecognized initially and taken to be early morning clumsiness. In approximately 80% of cases, generalized tonic-clonic seizures also occur, usually months or years after the onset of myoclonus, and it is these which often trigger the diagnosis. It is worth inquiring specifically about myoclonus in anyone presenting with generalized epilepsy. The tonic-clonic seizures are usually infrequent (average two a year). Approximately one-third of patients also develop typical absence seizures (usually very brief 2–5s) and again usually on awakning. Almost invariably, the absence seizures occur in patients with both myoclonus and tonic-clonic seizures. Approximately 5% of patients exhibit strong photosensitivity, and the myoclonus (and other seizures) can be precipitated by photic stimuli. The background EEG is normal. The good prognosis of this condition has been recognized since the 1920s. Complete response to treatment can be expected in 80%–90% of cases, but lifelong therapy can be needed. A family history of epilepsy is found in approximately 25% of cases, and in approximately 5% of close relatives (of whom one-third have JME, and most of the others have other IGE subtypes). The risk of epilepsy in offspring is approximately 5%.

EEG = electroencephalogram.

2.3.2 **Benign partial Epilepsy with Centrotemporal Spikes (BECTS) (Box 2.9)**

This condition (synonym: *Rolandic Epilepsy, Benign Epilepsy with Rolandic Spikes*) is the most common idiopathic localization-related epilepsy syndrome, accounting for perhaps 15% of all epilepsies. In the core syndrome, the peak age of onset is 5–8yrs and over 80% of cases have onset between 4yrs and –10yrs. The seizures are infrequent—25% of cases have only a single attack and 50% approximately five attacks in all. Less than 20% of cases have 20 or more seizures, and the total duration of seizure activity is 3 or more years in only 10%. Approximately 50% of children have seizures only at night, approximately 40% both in day and night, and in 10% seizures exclusively during the day. The seizures begin with spasm and clonic jerking of one side of the face and throat muscles. In many cases, the seizures sometimes evolve to secondarily generalized tonic-clonic attacks. The motor features may include speech arrest, a gurgling or guttural sound, and profuse salivation. The EEG shows focal spikes that originate most often in the centrotemporal regions.

Box 2.9 Benign partial Epilepsy with Centrotemporal Spikes (BECTS)

- 15% of all childhood epilepsy
- Age of onset 5–10yrs
- Simple partial seizures with frequent secondary generalization
- Partial seizures involve the face, oropharynx, and upper limb
- Seizures typically during sleep and infrequent
- No other neurological features; normal intelligence
- Family history sometimes present
- EEG shows typical centrotemporal spikes
- Excellent response to antiepileptic drugs
- Excellent prognosis with remission usual by mid-teenage years.

The prognosis of the typical condition is excellent and neurological development and cognitive function are generally normal and the seizures remit in more than 95% of cases. In a small number of cases, the epilepsy evolves into other more serious syndromic forms of epilepsy.

2.3.3 **Febrile seizures (Box 2.10)**

Febrile seizures are included in the category of 'situation-related seizures' of the ILAE classification. They are defined as epileptic events that occur in the context of an acute rise in body temperature, usually in children between 6 months and 6yrs of age, in whom there is no evidence of intracranial infection or other defined intrac-

EEG = electroencephalogram.

ranial cause. They are common: approximately 3%–5% of children will have at least one attack (7% in Japan), and it has been estimated that between 19 and 41/1,000 infants with fever will convulse. The first febrile seizure happens in the second year of life in 50% and in the first 3yrs in 90%. Four percent occur before 6 months and 6% after 6yrs. Febrile seizures are slightly more common in males. Febrile seizures are usually subdivided into simple and complex forms. Complex febrile seizures are those that last more than 15min or have strongly unilateral features. Up to one-third of all febrile convulsions are classifiable as complex.

The essentially benign simple febrile seizures need to be differentiated from the 5%–10% of first seizures with fever in which the seizure is in fact due to viral or bacterial meningitis and other cases where the fever lights up an existing latent predisposition to epilepsy. In neither of these situations should the 'febrile convulsion' be used, as both carry significantly different clinical implications.

Box 2.10 Febrile convulsions

- 2%–5% of all children
- Peak age of onset 2–5yrs
- 10%–20% of children have existing neurodevelopmental problems
- Convulsive seizures, sometimes with focal features. Can be prolonged in a minority of cases
- Usually at onset of fever
- 35% of children have a second febrile seizure and 15% a third (recurrence more likely with early age of onset, positive family history)
- Prognosis worse in complex febrile seizures (prolonged or focal; 30% of all febrile seizures) or young onset seizures

---

Approximately 35% of susceptible children will have a second febrile seizure and 15% three or more. The main risks associated with febrile seizures are of the development of hippocampal sclerosis and/or the development of subsequent epilepsy. These risks are increased if the seizures are complex and particularly if they are prolonged (Table 2.3). It is for this reason that febrile seizures should be treated as an emergency and urgent parenteral therapy given for any seizure lasting more than 5min. In a first febrile seizure, the infant should be taken urgently to hospital for evaluation to exclude underlying meningitis or cerebral disease.

Table 2.3 Prognosis of febrile seizures

	Simple febrile seizures (%)	Complex febrile seizures (%)	All febrile seizures (%)
Mortality	0	1.6	0.85
Risk of subsequent epilepsy	<6	10–20	2–7.5
Acute MRI changes	0	38.5	Not known
Hippocampal sclerosis on long-term follow-up	0	2.6	<1

MRI = magnetic resonance imaging.

2.3.4 West syndrome (Box 2.11)

West syndrome (synonym: Infantile Spasm) is a form of epileptic encephalopathy with an incidence of 0.25–0.42/1,000 live births and with a family history is 7%–17%. It is classified as a form of symptomatic or cryptogenic generalized epilepsy. The condition is defined by the occurrence of a typical form of epileptic seizure (the infantile spasm) and EEG change (hypsarrhythmia). Infantile spasms take the form of a sudden, generally bilateral, and symmetrical contractions of the muscles of the neck, trunk, or limbs. The spasms grow in frequency as the condition evolves, and at its peak, seizures often occur hundreds of times a day. The spasms show a strong tendency to cluster, with intensity waxing and waning during the cluster. The peak age of onset is 4–6 months, and the spasms rarely develop before the age of 3 months. 90% develop in the first year of life. The EEG shows the characteristic pattern of hypsarrhythmia in its fully developed form. Modified EEG forms frequently occur. A wide variety of conditions have been reported to cause this encephalopathy, of which the most common are as follows: tuberous sclerosis (7%–25% of all cases); neonatal ischaemia and infections (approximately 15% of all cases); lissencephaly and pachygyria and hemi-egalencephaly (approximately 10% of cases); and Down syndrome and acquired brain insults. West syndrome has a terrible position amongst the childhood epilepsies because of its severe prognosis in terms of seizure recurrence and mental development, rapid deterioration of psychomotor status, and resistance to conventional antiepileptic drug treatment. Treatment is with vigabatrin, which seems to be the conventional antiepileptic drug with the most marked effect in this condition, or with tetracosactide (adrenocorticotropic hormone (ACTH)) or corticosteroid treatment. On treatment, the spasms remit in almost all cases with few cases having attacks after the age of 3yrs. However, both the development of the child and the ultimate neurological status are usually impaired. 70%–96% of the survivors have learning difficulty (which in over 50% is severe) and in 35%–60% chronic epilepsy develops. The epilepsy can be severe, and evolve into the Lennox–Gastaut syndrome.

Box 2.11 **West syndrome**

- 1–2 cases per 4,000 live births
- Onset 4–8 months
- An age-specific epileptic encephalopathy
- Seizures take the form of infantile spasms (Salaam attacks)
- 20% cryptogenic, 80% symptomatic. Causes include neonatal and infantile infections, hypoxic-ischaemic encephalopathy, tuberous sclerosis, cortical dysplasia, chromosomal disorders, inherited metabolic disorders
- EEG shows hypsarrhythmia pattern
- Response to corticosteroids or vigabatrin
- Prognosis poor. 5% die in acute phase. Learning disability and continuing epilepsy are common sequels

2.3.5 **Lennox–Gastaut syndrome (Box 2.12)**

This term denotes an ill-defined age-specific epileptic encephalopathy with a wide range of causes. Although it remains a common view that this is a specific syndrome, some authorities disagree and view the clinical and EEG patterns as simply a reflection of severe epilepsy in childhood associated with learning disability. In favour of the latter view is the fact that there are many underlying causes, that there is no specific histopathology or specific treatment, and that the clinical pattern can evolve from other epilepsy syndromes (West syndrome, neonatal convulsions). Lennox–Gastaut syndrome accounts for between 1% and 5% of all childhood epilepsies, and occurs in up to 15% of institutionalized patients with mental handicap. The age of onset is between 1yr and 7yrs usually, although apparent adult-onset cases are recorded. In approximately 40% of cases, no cause is identifiable (these cases are termed cryptogenic Lennox–Gastaut syndrome). Approximately one-third of cases are due to malformations of brain development.

The epilepsy is very severe, with seizures often occurring many times a day. These take the form of atypical absence, tonic, myoclonic, tonic and tonic-clonic seizures, and later complex partial and other seizure types develop. The most characteristic seizure type is the tonic seizure. Nonconvulsive status (atypical absence status) may last hours or days and be repeated on an almost daily basis. Consciousness may be little affected in these periods (which can be referred to by carers as 'off days') although the patients are usually obtunded to some extent, and there may be additional signs, such as alteration of muscle tone, myoclonic jerks, or increased sialorrhea. The EEG signature of the condition is the presence interictally of long bursts of diffuse

EEG = electroencephalogram.

slow (1–2.5Hz) spike-wave activity, widespread in both hemispheres, roughly bilaterally synchronous but often asymmetrical. Learning disability is the other major feature of the condition. The intellectual impairment may be profound and at least 50% of cases have an intelligence quotient (IQ) below 50. There may be a slow deterioration in skills, although usually the condition is not progressive and sometimes better control of the epilepsy is usually possible by the time the sufferer reaches early adult life and this can result in intellectual improvement.

Box 2.12 Lennox–Gastaut syndrome

- 1%–5% of all childhood epilepsies
- Onset 1–14yrs
- Age-specific epileptic encephalopathy
- 40% 'cryptogenic', 60% symptomatic. Causes include cortical dysgenesis, neonatal, and infantile infection; ischaemic-hypoxic injury; tuberous sclerosis; Sturge–Weber syndrome; inherited metabolic disorders; chromosomal disorders
- Some cases evolve from West syndrome
- Learning disability—sometimes severe
- Multiple seizure types—atypical absence, tonic, atonic, tonic-clonic, myoclonic
- Episodes of nonconvulsive status epilepticus (75% of patients)
- Seizures precipitated by sedation and lack of stimulation
- Characteristic EEG pattern—slow spike-wave (≤2.5Hz), abnormal background, bursts of fast (≥10Hz) activity in non-REM sleep
- Poor response to antiepileptic therapy and seizures remit in <5% of cases

---

2.3.6 Severe myoclonic epilepsy in infancy (Dravet syndrome)

Dravet syndrome is a rare idiopathic generalized epilepsy syndrome, with a frequency of only 1 case per 30,000—40,000 children, but is mentioned here as it is one of the few epileptic encephalopathies which seems to result from a clear cut genetic abnormality, and one of the few with a rather specific treatment. Most cases have nonsense mutations or microdeletions or duplications of the *SCN1A* gene. The condition presents between 2 and 9 months of age taking the form of tonic-clonic or clonic seizures and often prolonged episodes of convulsive or nonconvulsive status epilepticus often provoked by fever. As the condition progresses, myoclonic, atypical absence, and

EEG = electroencephalogram.

partial seizures occur, and the patients develop ataxia, hyperactivity, and mental retardation. Conventional antiepileptic drug therapy does not control the seizures and lamotrigine may make them worse. One drug, stiripentol, seems to have a specific action in this condition and is licensed only for this condition. Topiramate is also helpful in some patients.

2.3.7 Generalized epilepsy with febrile seizures plus (GEFS+)

This is another epilepsy syndrome (included in the idiopathic generalized category) which although rare is one which has an interesting genetic basis. It is an autosomal dominant epilepsy syndrome in which defects in the *SCN1A*, *SCN1B*, and *GABRG2* genes have been found in different families (and in other families no identifiable genetic change). The syndrome is characterized by the occurrence of generalized (or partial) seizures, usually first occurring with fever, but later as afebrile seizures. Intelligence is usually normal, but varying degrees of learning disability can occur. Prognosis is variable. Whether this is really a single syndrome is doubtful, in view of the great variability of clinical form and genetic background.

2.3.8 Neonatal seizures

The neonatal period is defined as the first 28 days of life in a term infant or in premature infants, the period until gestational age of 44wks. Seizures occur in approximately 0.1% of neonates. Neonatal seizures are categorized in ILAE classification as an 'Epilepsy-uncertain whether focal or generalized'. Most neonatal seizures occur for a few days only, and <50% of affected infants develop long-term epilepsy. The clinical form of the seizures is very variable. The seizures can be very fragmentary and need to be differentiated from 'jitteryness', some are clearly focal and others multi-focal. The underlying cause determines prognosis.

The commonest cause is *hypoxic-ischemic encephalopathy* with seizures presenting in the first 72hrs of life. Intracranial haemorrhage is a common cause, especially in premature infants and subarachnoid haemorrhage in term infants. Metabolic disturbances which cause seizures include hypoglycaemia, hypocalcemia, and hypomagnesemia. Inborn errors of metabolism can present as neonatal seizures, usually when the infant begins to feed. Intracranial infections are an important and treatable cause of neonatal seizures. Bacterial meningitis with pathogens, which include *Escherichia coli* and *Streptococcus pneumoniae*, are an important cause. Major or severe cortical malformations can present with neonatal seizures.

There are several benign forms of neonatal epilepsy syndromes. *Benign familial neonatal convulsions* (second day seizures) which typically occur in the first 48–72hrs of life and disappear spontaneously by the age of 6 months. There is usually a family history and development is typically normal. A defect in the *KCNQ2* gene is often found. *Benign (nonfamilial) neonatal seizures* (fifth day seizures) typically present between day 4 and 6 of life. The cause has not been established but this form of epilepsy also has a generally excellent prognosis.

References and further reading

Arzimanoglou A, Guerrini R, and Aicardi J (2003). *Aicardi's epilepsy in children*, 3rd edn. Lippincott Williams & Wilkins, Philadelphia.

Engel J and Pedley TA (eds). (2007). *Epilepsy: a comprehensive textbook*, 3rd edn. Raven Press, New York.

Panayiotopoulos CP (2005). *The epilepsies: seizures, syndromes and management.* Bladon Medical Publisher, Chipping Norton.

Panayiotopoulos CP (2007). *A clinical guide to epileptic syndromes and their treatment.* Springer, New York.

Shorvon SD (2005). The clinical forms and causes of epilepsy. In SD Shorvon, ed. *Handbook of epilepsy treatment*, 2nd edn.. Blackwell Science, Oxford.

Shorvon SD (2009). The causes of epilepsy. In SD Shorvon, E Perucca, and J Engel, eds. *Treatment of epilepsy.* Wiley Blackwell, Oxford.

Wallace SJ and Farrell K (eds). (2004). *Epilepsy in children.* Arnold, London.

Chapter 3

The causes of epilepsy

> **Key points**
>
> - The cause of epilepsy is often multifactorial. In many cases, epilepsy is the result of a complex interaction of genetic and environmental factors.
> - Most diseases affecting the cerebral grey matter can result in epilepsy.
> - Approximately 10%–30% of all epilepsies are likely to have a predominantly genetic cause, although many genes are probably involved. In a small number of cases, a single genetic cause can be identified.
> - Congenital causes account for approximately 10% of cases.
> - The commonest acquired causes of epilepsy are vascular, tumoural, post-traumatic, or post-infectious. Hippocampal sclerosis is a cause of epilepsy in approximately 5%–10% of cases.
> - In approximately 30% of cases, no cause can be identified—these cases are referred to as 'cryptogenic epilepsy'.

Epilepsy is often multifactorial. Even when a major cause is identifiable (for instance, stroke or head injury), other factors (genetic and environmental) are often involved in the clinical manifestations (Table 3.1).

The range of aetiology varies in different age groups. Broadly speaking, congenital and perinatal conditions are the most common causes of early childhood onset epilepsy, whereas in adult life, epilepsy is more likely to be due to external non-genetic causes, but this distinction is by no means absolute. In late adult life, vascular disease is increasingly common. In certain parts of the world, endemic infections are common causes—including TB, cysticercosis, human immunodeficiency virus (HIV), and viral diseases.

Table 3.1 Approximate frequency of different causes of epilepsy	
Cause	**Approximate frequency (%)**
Idiopathic (probably polygenic)	10–30
Vascular	10–20
Congenital	5–10
Neurodegenerative/other neurological disorder	5–10
Hippocampal sclerosis	5–10
Brain tumour	5–10
Trauma	5
Childhood epilepsy syndrome	5
Infectious and post-infectious	5
Toxic and metabolic disorders	5
Single gene disorder	1–2
Unknown cause (cryptogenic epilepsy)	30

3.1 Epilepsy due to genetic or developmental causes

Heredity has an important influence on epilepsy, but the mechanisms are complex. Gene expression can be variable and influenced by environmental factors, and is often age dependent. The genetic influences are usually due to a complex interaction of many genes, and single gene disorders probably underlie only 1%–2% of all epilepsies. It is helpful to divide the genetic epilepsies into the following categories:

3.1.1 Pure epilepsies due to single gene disorders

These are inherited epilepsies in which epilepsy is the only or at least the major clinical feature. These are very rare conditions, described in families (sometimes single families) but are potentially important for the mechanistic light they may throw on the more common polygenic epilepsies. All the 13 genes identified to date (with one exception), which contribute to susceptibility to pure epilepsy, are genes that code for ion channel proteins.

3.1.2 Pure epilepsies with complex (presumed polygenic) inheritance

These are far more common than the single gene epilepsies. Categories of idiopathic and cryptogenic epilepsy, both focal and generalized, that exist have a strong presumption of a polygenic genetic basis (i.e. with complex inheritance, which does not follow simple Mendelian rules). These conditions include the *Idiopathic Generalized Epilepsies*

(IGE) and the *Benign Partial Epilepsies of Childhood*, and both have been the subject of intensive genetic study, but to date no common susceptibility genes have been identified. To what extent other cryptogenic epilepsies have a genetic basis is less clear (e.g. febrile convulsions, cryptogenic *West syndrome*, cryptogenic *Lennox–Gastaut syndrome*). The conditions are probably best conceptualized as polygenic disorders in which the phenotype is the result of interactions between susceptibility genes and environmental effects.

3.1.3 Other single gene disorders that have epilepsy as part of the phenotype

There are at least 240 single gene and chromosomal disorders resulting in neurological disorders in which epilepsy is part of the phenotype. Most are rare or very rare, manifest initially in childhood. In only a few of these conditions—for instance, the *Progressive Myoclonus Epilepsies* or the neurocutaneous syndromes—does the epilepsy have distinctive features, or is a predominant or consistent feature.

These conditions include the *inborn errors of metabolism* which are biochemical defects inherited usually in an autosomal recessive fashion, and in which the epilepsy is one symptom within a much broader spectrum of learning disability, neurological, and systemic features (Box 3.1).

Box 3.1 Some inborn errors of metabolism causing epilepsy

- Argininosuccinic aciduria
- Carnitine palmitoyltransferase 11 deficiency
- Glucocerebrosidase deficiency (Gaucher's disease)
- Hexosaminidase A deficiency
- Isovaleric acidaemia
- Mucopolysaccharidoses
- Neuronal ceroid lipofuscinoses
- Niemann–Pick disease
- Ornithine transcarbamylase deficiency
- Peroxisomal enzyme deficiencies
- Phenylalanine hydroxylase deficiency (phenylketonuria)
- Pyridoxine deficiency
- Pyruvate dehydrogenase deficiency
- Sialidoses
- Urea cycle disorders

The term *Progressive Myoclonic Epilepsy* (PME) is used to describe a rather specific phenotype which is the result of several different genetic disorders. In most parts of the world, there are six common underlying conditions that cause this syndrome: mitochondrial disorders (various types, including Alpers disease), Unverricht–Lundborg disease, dentate-rubro-pallido-luysian atrophy (DRLPA), Lafora body disease, neuronal ceroid lipofuscinosis, and sialidosis.

Neurocutaneous conditions are a group of genetically determined disorders which often result in epilepsy. Clinically, the most important are Tuberous Sclerosis Complex, Sturge–Weber syndrome, and Neurofibromatosis (type 1). Tuberous Sclerosis is a common and important cause of epilepsy and is usually caused by mutations of the *TSC1* or *TSC2* genes, both tumour suppression genes. In addition to epilepsy, there are a variety of other clinical abnormalities including characteristic skin lesions and other neurological, renal, and cardiac abnormalities. Neurofibromatosis (type 1: NF1) is another dominantly inherited genetic disorders, due to mutations in the *NF1* gene, occurring in approximately 1 in 3,000 live births. Almost half of all cases are new mutations. The epilepsy can take various forms including infantile spasms, partial and generalized seizures, and there are also characteristic skin and ophthalmic abnormalities. The genetic basis of Sturge–Weber syndrome has not been identified. The principle clinical features are a unilateral or bilateral port wine naevus, epilepsy, hemiparesis, mental impairment, and ocular signs.

3.1.4 **Epilepsy in disorders of chromosomal structure**

Epilepsy is also a feature of two common chromosomal abnormalities, *Down syndrome* and *Fragile X syndrome*. The rare condition *Ring Chromosome 20* manifests with a highly characteristic form of epilepsy, comprising long periods of nonconvulsive status epilepticus. Other uncommon chromosomal abnormalities in which epilepsy is part include *trisomy 12p, 8, 13, ring chromosome 14, partial monosomy 4p (Wolf–Hirschhorn syndrome), inverted duplication of peri-centromeric chromosome 15, and Klinefelter syndrome.*

3.1.5 **Epilepsies due to malformations of cortical development (cortical dysplasias)**

Cortical dysplasia (synonyms: cortical dysgenesis, malformations of cortical development) is a term which is applied to developmental disorders of the cortex that result in subtle or gross structural changes. Some of these conditions are caused by identifiable genetic abnormalities and others by environmental influences, such as infection, trauma, hypoxia, and exposure to drugs or toxins. In most cases, however, the cause is unclear. The forms of dysplasia consequent on environmental insults depend not only on the nature of the insult but also crucially on the stage of development at which the insult occurred.

The true prevalence of these conditions, previously thought to be rare, has only become apparent with the widespread use of magnetic resonance imaging (MRI) which has rendered cortical dysplasia visible in cases that were previously classified as cryptogenic. Examples of MRI images of cortical dysplasia are shown in Figures 3.1 and 3.2. Epilepsy is a leading feature of these conditions, usually but not always in association with learning disability and other neurological findings. The various categories of cortical dysplasia are shown in Box 3.2. The genes underlying many of these conditions are now identified (including defects in the *FLNA* gene (periventricular heterotopia), 6 genes for polymicrogyria, *DCX* gene (band heterotopia and lissencephaly), *LIS1* gene (lissencephaly), *RELN* and *ARX* genes, etc.).

Box 3.2 Types of cortical dysplasia

Abnormalities of gyration
Lissencephaly, macrogyria, pachygyria, polymicrogyria, schizencephaly, minor gyral abnormalities

Heterotopias
Subependymal nodular heterotopia, subcortical nodular heterotopia, subcortical band heterotopia

Other gross malformations
Megalencephaly and hemimegalencephaly, agenesis of corpus callosum, anencephaly and holoprosencephaly, microcephaly

Cortical dysgenesis associated with neoplasia
Dysembryoneuroepithelial tumour (DNET), ganglioglioma, gangliocytoma, hypothalamic hamartoma

Other cortical dysplasia
Focal cortical dysplasia, tuberous sclerosis microdysgenesis

Figure 3.1 **MRI scan showing subependymal heterotopia (arrowed)**

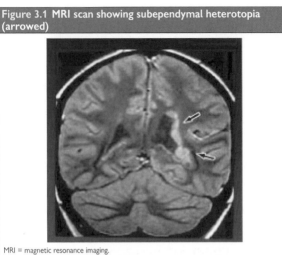

MRI = magnetic resonance imaging.

Figure 3.2 **MRI scans showing polymicrogyria. Reformatted surface-rendered (*top*) and axial (*bottom*) displays**

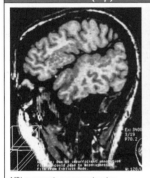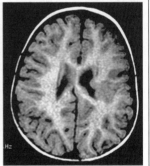

MRI = magnetic resonance imaging.

3.2 **Epilepsies due to acquired causes (the symptomatic epilepsies)**

Almost any condition affecting the cerebral grey matter can result in epilepsy, but here only the more common forms of acquired epilepsy will be mentioned. The investigation of cases will depend on the suspected cause, but in general terms, an accurate medical history is more important than any single test and will point to a presumptive diagnosis in most cases. Investigations which may be necessary range from MRI imaging, other neurological investigations such as cerebrospinal fluid (CSF) analysis, EEG and other biochemical, haematological, immunological, endocrinological, and histological examinations.

3.2.1 **Hippocampal sclerosis**

This term is used to describe the pathological lesion that comprises scarring, shrinkage, synaptic reorganization, and cell loss in the mesial temporal structures. It is the commonest cause of temporal lobe epilepsy, and is detected in approximately one-third of cases of people with refractory focal epilepsy attending hospital clinics in whom there is no other structural lesion (an example of MRI of the hippocampus is shown in Figure 3.3). The pathogenesis is probably multifactorial. There is a very clear association with a history of childhood febrile convulsions, and it is commonly believed that the lesion is the result of damage induced by prolonged or complex febrile seizures. There is also evidence that in some cases, hippocampal sclerosis may be a congenital lesion. Hippocampal sclerosis can also result from head injury and viral encephalitis. The epilepsy caused by hippocampal sclerosis typically takes the form of complex partial seizures of mesial temporal type with or without secondarily generalized seizures. The onset of the epilepsy depends on the cause, but is typically in childhood or early adult life. Hippocampal sclerosis can accompany other congenital lesions and especially cortical dysplasia (resulting in what is sometimes tagged as 'dual pathology'). Hippocampal sclerosis is sometimes bilateral, especially if the result of viral encephalitis. The outcome of unilateral temporal lobectomy is much less good in the presence of dual pathology or bilateral hippocampal sclerosis, and so both should be carefully sought as part of the pre-surgical workup.

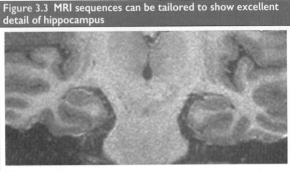

Figure 3.3 **MRI sequences can be tailored to show excellent detail of hippocampus**

MRI = magnetic resonance imaging.

3.2.2 **Prenatal or perinatal injury**

Epilepsy has traditionally often been thought to occur due to perinatal injury, although it is now recognized that many such cases have in fact genetic or other prenatal developmental pathologies causing the epilepsy. In controlled studies, only severe perinatal insults have been found to increase the risk of subsequent epilepsy—for instance, perinatal haemorrhage, ischaemic–hypoxic encephalopathy. Factors such as toxaemia, eclampsia, forceps delivery, being born with the 'cord round the neck', low birth rate, or prematurity have only a very modest association, if any, with subsequent epilepsy.

3.2.3 **Post-vaccination encephalitic encephalomyelitis**

The possible role of vaccination (particularly pertussis vaccination) in causing a childhood encephalopathy and subsequent epilepsy and learning disability has been the subject of intense study, with contradictory claims. There is a fairly general consensus now that the risk of vaccine-induced encephalopathy and/or epilepsy, if it exists at all, is extremely low. Risk estimates in the literature have included risk of a febrile seizure 1 per 19,496 pertussis vaccinations; risk of an afebrile seizure 1 per 76,133 vaccinations; and risk of encephalopathy after pertussis infection nil-3 cases per million vaccinations. Some cases of apparent vaccination injury are in fact due to the presence of an inherited genetic defect of the *SCNIA* gene, which is the root cause of the epilepsy.

3.2.4 **Post-traumatic epilepsy**

Head trauma is an important cause of epilepsy. It is customary to draw a distinction between open head injury, where the dura is breached, and closed head injury, where there is no dural breach. Post-traumatic seizures are traditionally subdivided into immediate, early, and late categories. Immediate seizures are defined as those that occur within the first 24hr after injury, early seizures are those that occur within the first week, and late seizures are those that occur after 1wk. Approximately 5% of all those admitted to hospital with head injury experience early seizures, and they are more common in children than adults.

Closed head injuries are commonest in civilian practice, usually from road traffic accidents, falls, or recreational injuries, and in different series have accounted for between 2% and 12% of all cases of epilepsy. In mild head injury—defined as head injury without skull fracture and with less than 30min of post-traumatic amnesia—there is no marked increased risk of epilepsy. Moderate head injury—defined as a head injury complicated by skull fracture and/or post-traumatic amnesia for more than 30min—is followed by epilepsy in approximately 1%–4% of cases. Severe head injury—defined as a head injury with post-traumatic amnesia of more than 24hr, intracranial haematoma or cerebral contusion—has been found in most studies to be followed by epilepsy in 10% or more of patients. In a recent very large population-based study, the relative risk for epilepsy was 2.22 (95% CI 2.07–2.38) in the presence of mild brain injury and 7.40 (95% CI 6.16-8.89) in the presence of severe brain injury.

Open head injury is a more potent cause of epilepsy. Between 30% and 50% of patients in penetrating wartime injuries suffer subsequent epilepsy.

Overall, the risk of late epilepsy, if early epilepsy is present, is approximately 25% compared to 3% in patients who did not have early seizures. In patients admitted to hospital, the risk of late epilepsy is approximately 35% if there is an intracranial haematoma and approximately 5% if not, and approximately 17% if there is a depressed skull facture and 4% if not. If there is neither haematoma nor depressed skull fracture, the risk of epilepsy is 1% if there were no early seizures and 26% if there were early seizures.

3.2.5 Epilepsy due to brain tumours

Brain tumours are responsible for approximately 5%–10% of all newly diagnosed cases of epilepsy. The rate is greatest in adults, and approximately one-quarter of adults presenting with newly developing focal epilepsy have an underlying tumour, compared to less than 5% in children. The frequency of seizures is high in tumours in the frontal, central, and temporal regions; lower in posterior cortically placed tumours; and very low in subcortical tumours. Epilepsy occurs in 92% of those with oligodendrogliomas, 70% of those with astrocytomas and 37% of those with glioblastomas. Epilepsy is the first symptom of meningioma in 20%–50% of cases. In slow growing tumours, the history of epilepsy will often have extended for decades, sometimes even into infancy.

In chronic refractory tumoural epilepsy, oligodendrogliomas account for between 10% and 40% of cases, dysembryoplastic neuroepithelial tumours (DNETs) for 10%–30%, astrocytomas for 10%–30%, and gangliogliomas or hamartomas each for between 10% and 20%.

Hypothalamic hamartomas are a rare tumour, but one with a characteristic phenotype. They usually present in young children with gelastic seizures, learning disability, behavioural disturbance, and later with precocious puberty.

3.2.6 **Epilepsy following cerebral infection**

3.2.6.1 *Meningitis and encephalitis*

The risk of chronic epilepsy following encephalitis or meningitis is almost sevenfold greater than that in the population. The increased risk is highest during the first 5yrs after infection, but remains elevated for up to 15yrs. The risk is much higher after encephalitis (RR 16.2) than bacterial meningitis (RR 4.2) or aseptic meningitis (RR 2.3).

The commonest serious viral encephalitis is due to HSV-1 and this frequently results in severe and intractable epilepsy. The incidence of severe HSV-1 encephalitis is approximately 2 per million persons per year (about 10–20% of all cases of viral encephalitis).

3.2.6.2 *Cerebral malaria*

Seizures and typically status epilepticus are particularly common in the acute phase of cerebral malaria, and there is a 9–11 (CI 2-18) fold increase in risk of chronic epilepsy in children with a history of malaria.

3.2.6.3 *Pyogenic cerebral abscess*

Pyogenic brain abscess is an uncommon but serious cause of infective epilepsy. Commonly isolated organisms are streptococci, including aerobic, anaerobic, and microaerophilic types. *Streptococcus pneumoniae* is a rarer cause of brain abscesses and sometimes the sequel to occult cerebrospinal fluid (CSF) rhinorrhoea, and also to pneumococcal pneumonia in elderly patients. Enteric bacteria and *Bacteroides* are isolated in 20%–40% of cases and often in mixed culture. Staphylococcal abscesses account for 10%–15% of cases and are usually caused by penetrating head injury or bacteraemia secondary to endocarditis. Clostridial infections are most often post-traumatic. Very rarely, brain abscess can be caused by fungi such as *Actinomyces* or *Nocardia*.

3.2.6.4 *Neurocysticercosis*

Worldwide, neurocysticercosis (NCC) is the most common parasitic disease of the central nervous system (CNS) and a major cause of epilepsy in endemic areas such as Mexico, India, and China. The condition is a helminthiasis caused by the encysted larval stage, *Cysticercus cellulosae*, of the pork tapeworm *Taenia solium*. In the first stage, the human (definitive) host ingests undercooked diseased pork containing viable cysticerci, which grow into tapeworms in the human gut. Eggs are released into the faeces and hatch in the pig (intermediate host). Humans become intermediate hosts by ingesting infected tissue, and the cysts migrate to the human CNS, skin, and muscle. The brain cysts can be single or multiple. Epilepsy is the commonest clinical manifestation and usual presenting feature of NCC. Diagnosis is made by imaging and by serological tests. CSF and electroencephalogram (EEG) are rather non-specific. Newer enzyme-linked immuno-electron transfer blot (EITB) assays on CSF or serum appear to have higher sensitivity (98%) and specificity (100%) in multiple cysticercosis. Recently, an antigen detection ('direct capture') immunoassay specific for viable metacestodes in CSF has been designed.

3.2.6.5 *Tuberculoma*

Epilepsy is frequently the presenting symptom of tuberculoma. Tuberculoma accounts for approximately 3% of all cerebral mass lesions in India, for instance, and 13% of all cerebral lesions in HIV-infected patients. Diagnosis depends on the clinical context, imaging, serology, and histological examination of biopsy material.

3.2.6.6 *Rasmussen's encephalitis*

This rare progressive disorder presents as focal epilepsy and unilateral hemiplegia and/or other symptoms of unilateral cortical dysfunction. The cause is unknown although viral causes have been implicated in some cases. Diagnosis is on the basis of the clinical and MRI findings.

3.2.7 **Epilepsy due to cerebrovascular disease**

Epilepsy can complicate all forms of cerebrovascular disease. Stroke is the most commonly identified cause of epilepsy in the elderly, and occult stroke also explains the occurrence of many cases of apparently cryptogenic epilepsies in aged individuals. A history of stroke has been found to be associated with an increased lifetime occurrence of epilepsy (OR 3.3; 95% CI 1.3–8.5). Status epilepticus occurs in the acute phase of approximately 1% of all strokes, and 20% of status epilepticus is due to stroke.

3.2.7.1 *Cerebral haemorrhage*

The reported risk of chronic epilepsy due to intracranial haemorrhage has varied greatly from series to series, but is generally in the region of 10%. Epilepsy is more common after large haemorrhages and haemorrhages that involve the cerebral cortex, and less common in deep haematomas and rare after subtentorial haemorrhage. The epilepsy almost always develops within 2yrs of the haemorrhage. The risk of seizures after subarachnoid haemorrhage is between 20% and 34%.

3.2.7.2 *Cerebral infarction*

Epilepsy occurs in approximately 6% of patients within 12 months and 11% within 5yrs of a stroke due to cerebral infarction. The risk of epilepsy is approximately 17–20 times than in non-stroke controls.

Factors associated with a greater risk of epilepsy have been the subject of several studies, and are as follows: severity, size of infarct, haemorrhagic transformation, a cortical (as opposed to subcortical) site of the stroke, and in some studies embolism as a cause of the stroke.

3.2.7.3 *Occult cerebrovascular disease*

Late-onset epilepsy can be the first manifestation of cerebrovascular disease. Between 5% and 10% of patients presenting with stroke have a history of prior epileptic seizures in the recent past, and in the absence of other causes, new-onset seizures should prompt a screen for vascular risk factors.

3.2.7.4 *Arteriovenous malformations*

Between 17% and 36% of supratentorial arteriovenous malformations (AVMs) present with seizures, with or without associated neurological deficits, and 40%–50% with haemorrhage. Smaller arterial AVMs (<3cm diameter) are more likely to present with haemorrhage than large ones. Conversely, large and/or superficial malformations are more epileptogenic, as are AVMs in the temporal lobe. Approximately 40% of patients with large anterior venous malformations have epilepsy, and epilepsy is the presenting symptom in approximately 20%. Small venous malformations do not usually result in any symptoms. The risk of haemorrhage from a venous angioma is lower than from an arterial angioma.

3.2.7.5 *Cavernous haemangioma*

These account for 5%–13% of vascular malformations of the CNS and are present in 0.02%–0.13% of autopsy series. Patients present with seizures (40%–70%), focal neurological deficits (35%–50%), non-specific headaches (10%–30%), and cerebral haemorrhage. Familial clustering can be found in 10%–30% of cavernous haemangiomas, and familial cases have been found to be linked to genes at three different loci, the *CCM1*, *CCM2*, and *CCM3* genes. Forty per cent of familial cases are due to *CCM1*, with higher rates amongst Hispanic cases. Genetic testing is available. The MRI appearances are characteristic.

3.2.7.6 *Other vascular disease*

Epilepsy can be a symptom of many other forms of vascular disease. Cortical venous infarcts are particularly epileptogenic, at least in the acute phase, and may underlie a significant proportion of apparently spontaneous epileptic seizures complicating other medical conditions and pregnancy for instance. Seizures also occur with cerebrovascular lesions secondary to rheumatic heart disease, endocarditis, mitral valve prolapse, cardiac tumours and cardiac arrhythmia, or after carotid endarterectomy. Infarction is also an important cause for seizures in neonatal epilepsy. Epilepsy is also common in eclampsia, hypertensive encephalopathy, and malignant hypertension, and in the anoxic encephalopathy which follows cardiac arrest or cardiopulmonary surgery.

Unruptured aneurysms occasionally present as epilepsy, especially if large and if embedded in the temporal lobe—for instance, a giant middle cerebral or anterior communicating aneurysm.

Epilepsy, with a vascular basis, also occurs in antiphospholipid syndrome, CADASIL, Moyamoya disease, collagen disease (e.g. Ehlers–Danlos, Marfan syndrome), vasculitis, Behçet's disease, and amyloid angiopathy. Other rare causes of epilepsy include temporal arteritis, polyarteritis nodosum, Takayasu disease, Fabry's disease, and the hyperviscosity syndrome.

3.2.8 Epilepsy in inflammatory and immunological diseases of the nervous system

3.2.8.1 *Demyelinating disorders*

The frequency of epilepsy in patients with multiple sclerosis (MS) is approximately three times that in the general population. In one study, the cumulative risk of epilepsy in patients with MS was found to be 1.1% at 5yrs, 1.8% by 10yrs, and 3.1% by 15yrs. Acute disseminated encephalomyelitis (ADEM) is an acute inflammatory demyelinating disorder which can follow systemic infections, and which is immunologically mediated. Epilepsy is a feature of the acute attack, and occurs much more commonly than in an acute attack of MS.

3.2.8.2 *Other CNS inflammatory and immunological disorders*

Epilepsy can occur in all other forms of large, medium, or small vessel vasculitis, sometimes on the basis of infarction. Seizures occur in approximately 25% of cases of *systemic lupus erythematosis*. Seizures can be the presenting symptom, and are particularly common in severe or chronic cases and in lupus-induced encephalopathy. Epilepsy occurs less often in other vasculitides such as Behçet's disease and in other 'connective tissue disorders' such as *Sjorgrens syndrome*, and mixed connective tissue disease and *Henoch-Schönlein purpura*. Seizures are the commonest neurological complication of the inflammatory bowel diseases (Ulcerative Colitis and Crohn's disease) occurring in one series in 6% of cases, and are a prominent feature of Hashimoto's thyroiditis, a relapsing encephalopathy associated with high titres of thyroid antibody. There has been recent interest in the occurrence of epilepsy in the syndrome of limbic encephalitis, associated with high titres of antibodies against voltage-gated potassium channels (VGKC). The epilepsy usually presents as a subacute illness, associated also with psychosis, neurological signs (e.g. ataxia), memory loss, and behavioural change. Other cases of limbic encephalitis have no detectable antibody present although in such cases the cause is likely to be an as yet unidentified antibody, and some are paraneoplastic.

3.2.9 **Reflex epilepsies**

The term reflex epilepsy is used to describe cases in which seizures are evoked consistently by a specific environmental trigger. The reflex epilepsies are sometimes subdivided into simple and complex types. In the simple forms, the seizures are precipitated by simple sensory stimuli (e.g. flashes of light; startle) and in the complex forms by more elaborate stimuli (e.g. specific pieces of music). The complex forms are much more heterogeneous and the syndromes are less well defined than the simple reflex epilepsies. In hospital practice, approximately 5% of patients show some features of reflex epilepsy. The stimuli most reported to cause seizures include flashing lights and other visual stimuli, startle, eating, hot water, music, reading, and movement.

The commonest reflex epilepsies are those induced by visual stimuli. Flashing lights, bright lights, moving visual patterns (e.g. escalators), eye closure, moving from dark into bright light, and viewing specific objects or colours have all been described to induce seizures. The term photosensitive epilepsy should be confined to those individuals who show unequivocal EEG evidence of photosensitivity, and differentiated from other, usually more complex, cases in which seizures can be apparently precipitated by visual stimuli but in whom EEG evidence of photosensitivity cannot be demonstrated. Photosensitivity (strictly defined) is present in a population with a frequency of approximately 1.1/100,000 persons, and 5.7/100,000 in the 7–19 age range, and very strongly associated with epilepsy. Approximately 3% of persons with epilepsy are photosensitive and have seizures induced by photic stimuli (usually viewing flickering or intermittent lights or cathode ray monitors, bright lights or repeating patterns). Most patients with photosensitivity have the syndrome of *IGE*, although photosensitivity is also occurs in patients with focal epilepsy arising in the occipital region and occasionally in other conditions (Box 3.3).

Box 3.3 **Epilepsies associated with photosensitivity**
Idiopathic generalized epilepsy*
Progressive myoclonic epilepsies
Focal occipital epilepsy
Mitochondrial diseases
Inborn errors of metabolism
Symptomatic generalized and localization-related epilepsy**
Idiopathic localization-related epilepsy**

* Idiopathic Generalized Epilepsy (IGE) is the most common form of photosensitive epilepsy.

** Photosensitivity is rare in idiopathic localization-related or symptomatic epilepsy.

3.2.10 **Metabolic and endocrine-induced seizures**

Many types of metabolic or endocrine disturbances can cause epilepsy. Hyponatraemia is the commonest electrolyte disturbance to result in epileptic seizures, which typically occur if the serum sodium falls below 115 mmol/L, although the rate of fall is an important variable—the faster the rate, the higher the chance of a seizure. Seizures also routinely occur in the presence of hypocalcaemia, hypercalcaemia, hypomagnesaemia, hypokalaemia, and hyperkalaemia. Ten per cent of patients with severe renal failure have seizures, caused either by the metabolic disturbance, renal encephalopathy, and dialysis encephalopathy or dialysis disequilibrium syndrome. Seizures are a common occurrence in hepatic failure. Hepatic encephalopathy may be overlooked and routine liver function tests can be relatively normal. Hyperammonaemia is sometimes diagnostically helpful in detecting liver disease and can be a cause of seizures. Reye's syndrome should be considered in patients with liver failure, especially children where it is associated with aspirin intake.

Hypoglycaemia is a potent cause of seizures—which can occur if the blood sugar levels fall below 2.2 mmol/L. This is commonly due to insulin therapy in patients with diabetes, but can also be due to insulinoma and to drugs such as quinine and pentamidine. Non-ketotic hyperglycaemia frequently causes seizures. Levels of blood sugar as low as 15–20 mmol/L can cause seizures if there is associated hyperosmolarity. The seizures in non-ketotic hyperglycaemia can be focal and this implies the presence of cerebral pathology (usually cerebrovascular disease). Diabetic ketoacidosis does not frequently result in seizures.

3.2.11 **Alcohol, toxin, and drug-induced seizures**

Alcohol abuse is a potent cause of epilepsy. Binge drinking can result in acute cerebral toxicity and seizures. Alcohol withdrawal in an alcohol-dependent person carries an even greater risk of seizures. Seizures can also be caused by the metabolic disturbances associated with binge drinking, the cerebral damage due to trauma, cerebral infection, subdural haematoma, the chronic neurotoxic effects of chronic alcohol exposure, or to acute Wernicke's encephalopathy due to thiamine deficiency.

Seizures can also be provoked by exposure to many different toxins. Potent causes include heavy metal poisoning, and carbon monoxide poisoning with carboxyhaemoglobin levels over 50%.

A wide range of drugs, toxins, and illicit compounds can cause acute symptomatic seizures and epilepsy (Box 3.4), although seizures accounted for less than 1% of 32,812 consecutive patients prospectively monitored for drug toxicity.

> **Box 3.4 Some drugs which can cause seizures**
>
> - Antipsychotic drugs
> - Antidepressant drugs
> - Narcotic analgesics
> - Infusional and inhalational anaesthetics
> - Anti-malarial drugs (especially mefloquine)
> - Cytoxic drugs
> - Theophylline
> - Anti-arrhythmic agents
> - Recreational and performance-enhancing drugs, for instance, cocaine, amphetamine. 'ecstasy' (3,4-methylenedioxy-methamphetamine (MDMA)), phencyclidine (angel dust), lysergic acid diethylamide (LSD), erythropoietin

References and further reading

Annegers JF, Hauser WA, Beghi E, Nicolosi A, and Kurland LT (1988). The risk of unprovoked seizures after encephalitis and meningitis. *Neurology*, **38**, 1407–10.

Annegers JF, Hauser WA, Lee JR, and Rocca WA (1995). Incidence of acute symptomatic seizures in Rochester, Minnesota, 1935–1984. *Epilepsia*, **36**, 327–33.

Annegers JF, Hauser WA, Coan SP, and Rocca WA (1998). A population-based study of seizures after traumatic brain injuries. *New England Journal of Medicine*, **338**, 20–4.

Baulac S, Gourfinkel-An I, Nabbout R, et al. (2004). Fever, genes, and epilepsy. *Lancet Neurology*, **3**, 421–30.

Bergamasco B, Benna P, Ferrero P, and Gavinelli R (1984). Neonatal hypoxia and epileptic risk: a clinical prospective study. *Epilepsia*, **25**, 131–6.

Berkovic SF, Harkin L, McMahon JM, et al. (2006). De-novo mutations of the sodium channel gene SCN1A in alleged vaccine encephalopathy: a retrospective study. *Lancet Neurology*, **5**, 488–92.

Burn J, Dennis M, Bamford J, Sandercock P, Wade D, and Warlow C (1997). Epileptic seizures after a first stroke: the Oxfordshire Community Stroke Project. *BMJ*, **315**, 1582–7.

Carpio A, Escobar A, and Hauser WA (1998). Cysticercosis and epilepsy: a critical review. *Epilepsia*, **39**, 1025–40.

Carter JA, Neville BG, White S, et al. (2004). Increased prevalence of epilepsy associated with severe falciparum malaria in children. *Epilepsia*, **45**, 978–81.

Cascino GD (1990). Epilepsy and brain tumors: implications for treatment. *Epilepsia*, **31** (Suppl 3) S37–44.

Castilla-Guerra L, del Carmen Fernández-Moreno M, López-Chozas JM, and Fernández-Bolaños R (2006). Electrolytes disturbances and seizures. *Epilepsia*, **47**, 1990–8.

Camilo O and Goldstein LB. (2004). Seizures and epilepsy after ischemic stroke. *Stroke*, **35**, 1769–75.

Cervoni L, Artico M, Salvati M, Bristot R, Franco C, and Delfini R (1994). Epileptic seizures in intracerebral hemorrhage: a clinical and prognostic study of 55 cases. *Neurosurgery Review*, **17**, 185–8.

Cimaz R, Meroni PL, and Shoenfeld Y (2006). Epilepsy as part of systemic lupus erythematosus and systemic antiphospholipid syndrome (Hughes syndrome). *Lupus*, **15**, 191–7.

Cleary P, Shorvon S, and Tallis R (2004). Late-onset seizures as a predictor of subsequent stroke. *Lancet*, **363**, 1184–6.

Crawford PM, West CR, Shaw MDM, and Chadwick DW (1986). Cerebral arteriovenous malformations and epilepsy: factors in the development of epilepsy. *Epilepsia*, **27**, 270–5.

Daumas-Duport C, Scheithauer BW, Chodkiewicz JP, Laws ER Jr, and Vedrenne C (1988). Dysembryoplastic neuroepithelial tumor: a surgically curable tumor of young patients with intractable partial seizures. Report of thirty-nine cases. *Neurosurgery*, **23**, 545–56.

Delanty N, Vaughan CJ, and French JA (1998). Medical causes of seizures. *Lancet*, **352**, 383–90.

Devlin RJ and Henry JA (2008). Clinical review: major consequences of illicit drug consumption. *Critical care (London, England)*, **12**, 202.

Dravet C, Bureau M, Oguni H, Fukuyama Y, and Cokar O (2005). Severe myoclonic epilepsy in infancy: Dravet syndrome. *Advances in Neurology*, **95**, 71–102.

Friedlander RM (2007). Clinical practice. Arteriovenous malformations of the brain. *The New England Journal of Medicine*, **356**, 2704–12.

Freeman JL, Coleman LT, Wellard RM, et al. (2004). MR imaging and spectroscopic study of epileptogenic hypothalamic hamartomas: analysis of 72 cases. *American Journal of Nephrology*, **25**, 450–62.

Gambardella A, Andermann F, Shorvon S, Le Piane E, and Aguglia U (2008). Limited chronic focal encephalitis: another variant of Rasmussen syndrome? *Neurology*, **70**, 374–7.

Garcia HH and Modi M (2008). Helminthic parasites and seizures. *Epilepsia*, **49**(Suppl 6), 25–32.

Gordon E and Devinsky O (2001). Alcohol and marijuana: effects on epilepsy and use by patients with epilepsy. *Epilepsia*, **42**, 1266–72.

Guerrini R and Marini C (2006). Genetic malformations of cortical development. *Experimental Brain Research*, **173**, 322–33.

Guerrini R, Carrozzo R, Rinaldi R, and Bonanni P. (2003). Angelman syndrome: etiology, clinical features, diagnosis, and management of symptoms. *Paediatric Drugs*, **5**, 647–61.

Guerrini R, Dobyns WB, and Barkovich AJ (2008). Abnormal development of the human cerebral cortex: genetics, functional consequences and treatment options. *Trends in Neurosciences*, **31**, 154–62.

Hillbom M, Pieninkeroinen I, and Leone M (2003). Seizures in alcohol-dependent patients: epidemiology, pathophysiology and management. *CNS Drugs*, **7**, 1013–30.

Hindmarsh JT (2003). The porphyrias, appropriate test selection. *Clinica Chimica Acta; International Journal of Clinical Chemistry*, **333**, 203–7.

Inoue Y, Fujiwara T, Matsuda K, et al. (1997). Ring chromosome 20 and nonconvulsive status epilepticus. A new epileptic syndrome. *Brain*, **120**(Pt 6), 939–53.

Joensuu T, Lehesjoki AE, and Kopra O (2008). Molecular background of EPM1-Unverricht-Lundborg disease. *Epilepsia*, **49**, 557–63.

Kälviäinen R, Khyuppenen J, Koskenkorva P, Eriksson K, Vanninen R, and Mervaala E (2008). Clinical picture of EPM1-Unverricht-Lundborg disease. *Epilepsia*, **49**(4), 549–56.

Kumar Garg R, Kumar Singh M, and Misra S (2000). Single-enhancing CT lesions in Indian patients with seizures: a review. *Epilepsy Research*, **38**, 91–104.

Lang B, Dale RC, and Vincent A (2003). New autoantibody mediated disorders of the central nervous system. *Current Opinion in Neurology*, **16**(3), 351–7.

Leventer RJ, Guerrini R, and Dobyns WB (2008). Malformations of cortical development and epilepsy. *Dialogues in Clinical Neuroscience*, 10(1), 47–62.

Marcotte L and Crino PB. (2006). The neurobiology of the tuberous sclerosis complex. *Neuromolecular Medicine*, **8**, 531–46.

Meinck HM (2006). Startle and its disorders. *Neurophysiologie Clinique*, **36**(5–6), 357–64.

Menéndez M (2005). Down syndrome, Alzheimer's disease and seizures. *Brain & Development*, **27**, 246–52.

Moran NF, Fish DR, Kitchen N, Shorvon S, Kendall BE, and Stevens JM (1999). Supratentorial cavernous haemangiomas and epilepsy: a review of the literature and case series. *Journal of Neurology, Neurosurgery, and Psychiatry*, **66**, 561–8.

Moreno A, de Felipe J, García Sola R, Navarro A, and Ramón y Cajal S (2001). Neuronal and mixed neuronal glial tumors associated to epilepsy. A heterogeneous and related group of tumours. *Histology and Histopathology*, **16**, 613–22.

Morse RP (2004). Rasmussen encephalitis. *Archives of Neurology*, **61**, 592–4.

Mturi N, Musumba CO, Wamola BM, Ogutu BR, and Newton CR (2003). Cerebral malaria: optimising management. *CNS Drugs*, **17**, 153–65.

Nelson KB and Ellenberg JH (1987). Predisposing and causative factors in childhood epilepsy. *Epilepsia*, **28**(Suppl 1), S16–24.

Olafsson E, Gudmundsson G, and Hauser WA (2000). Risk of epilepsy in long-term survivors of surgery for aneurysmal subarachnoid hemorrhage: a population-based study in Iceland. *Epilepsia*, **41**, 1201–5.

Panayiotopoulos CP (2004). *The epilepsies: seizures, syndromes and management*. Bladon Medical Publishing, London.

Rantakallio P and von Wendt L (1986). A prospective comparative study of the aetiology of cerebral palsy and epilepsy in a one-year birth cohort from Northern Finland. *Acta paediatrica Scandinavica,* **75**, 586–92.

Sáenz-Lope E, Herranz-Tanarro FJ, and Masdeu JC (1985). Primary reading epilepsy. *Epilepsia,* **26**, 649–56.

Satishchandra P and Sinha S (2008). Seizures in HIV-seropositive individuals: NINHAMS experience and review. *Epilepsia,* **49**(Suppl 6), 33–41.

Scheffer IE, Harkin LA, Grinton BE, et al. (2007). Temporal lobe epilepsy and GEFS+ phenotypes associated with SCN1B mutations. *Brain,* **130**, 100–9.

Sedel F, Gourfinkel-An I, Lyon-Caen O, Baulac M, Saudubray JM, and Navarro V (2007). Epilepsy and inborn errors of metabolism in adults: a diagnostic approach. *Journal of Inherited Metabolic Disease,* **30**(6), 846–54.

Singh R, Gardner RJ, Crossland KM, Scheffer IE, and Berkovic SF (2002). Chromosomal abnormalities and epilepsy: a review for clinicians and gene hunters. *Epilepsia,* **43**, 127–40.

Shorvon SD (1995). Epilepsy after head injury and intracranial surgery. In A Hopkins, SD Shorvon, G Cascino (eds), *Epilepsy.* Chapman and Hall Medical, London.

Shorvon SD (2009). The aetiology of epilepsy. In SD Shorvon, E Perucca, J Engel (eds), *The treatment of epilepsy.* Wiley Blackwell, Oxford.

Shorvon S and Berg A (2008). Pertussis vaccination and epilepsy—an erratic history, new research and the mismatch between science and social policy. *Epilepsia,* **49**, 219–25.

Teasell R, Bayona N, Lippert C, Villamere J, and Hellings C (2007). Post-traumatic seizure disorder following acquired brain injury. *Brain Injury,* **21**, 201–14.

Trenité DG (2006). Photosensitivity, visually sensitive seizures and epilepsies. *Epilepsy Research,* **70**(Suppl 1), S269–79.

Vincent A and Bien CG (2005). Temporal lobe seizures, amnesia and autoantibodies—identifying a potentially reversible form of non-paraneoplastic limbic encephalitis. *Epileptic Disorders,* **7**, 177–9.

47

Chapter 4

The differential diagnosis and investigation of epilepsy

Key points

- The differential diagnosis of epilepsy is wide. It is not uncommon for epilepsy to be misdiagnosed.
- The key to diagnosis is to obtain a good first hand witnessed account or a video of a seizure.
- The commonest conditions confused with epilepsy are syncope and non-epileptic attack disorder (NEAD; pseudoseizures). A wide range of other conditions also enter into the differential diagnosis.
- A positive electroencephalogram (EEG) is a useful confirmation of a diagnosis of epilepsy, but in new cases of epilepsy approximately 50% of routine EEGs are normal. EEG is often misinterpreted, and many patients have a misdiagnosis of epilepsy because of misinterpretation of their EEG.
- Magnetic resonance imaging (MRI) is useful for establishing the cause of epilepsy. Sensitivity is increased by tailoring the MRI sequences and scanning parameters to the clinical situation.

4.1 Differential diagnosis

Epilepsy is a feature of many different neurological diseases and can take many different forms. The key to a correct diagnosis is a detailed history from both the patient and a reliable witness. Misdiagnosis is common; in tertiary referral practice, it is estimated that in 20% of those with a diagnosis of refractory epilepsy the diagnosis is incorrect. A videotape recording of an episode is also invaluable. Video cameras, particularly on mobile telephones, make such recordings feasible.

The stereotyped nature of the attack is an important feature in considering the diagnosis. Other features seen in many cases are lack of obvious immediate precipitant, short duration, tendency to cluster, occurrence in both daytime and sleep, relationship to sleep deprivation and alcohol, and characteristic after effects.

Epileptic seizures can present in a number of different ways summarized in Box 4.1, and because of this, the differential diagnosis is wide.

The commonest conditions which can be confused with epilepsy are as follows:

4.1.1 **Syncope**

Syncope (fainting) is the condition most commonly mistaken as epilepsy. It is caused by a sudden and massive fall in cerebral blood flow (a very different situation from an epileptic seizure, in which cerebral blood flow increases). The fall in blood flow can be due to a systemic reflex (vaso-vagal syncope), respiratory effort resulting in a valsalva manoeuvre (respiratory syncope), a failure of cardiac output (cardiogenic syncope), and a failure of peripheral resistance (postural/neuropathic) (Box 4.2).

Box 4.1 Clinical presentations of epilepsy

- Loss of awareness
- Generalized convulsive movements
- Drop attacks
- Transient focal motor attacks
- Transient focal sensory attacks
- Facial muscle and eye movements
- Psychic experiences
- Aggressive or vocal outbursts
- Episodic phenomena in sleep
- Prolonged confusional or fugue states

Box 4.2 Types of syncope

Reflex (vaso-vagal)
Precipitated by such factors as venusection, pain, emotion, hot surroundings, upright posture, micturition

Cardiac
Rheumatic heart diseases (especially aortic stenosis), ischaemic heart disease, congenital heart disease, outflow obstruction, prolonged QT syndrome, other causes of dysrhythmia

Postural/neuropathic
Alcohol, drugs, old age, hypovolaemia, peripheral neuropathy (areflexic syncope), and autonomic failure

Respiratory (valsalva manoeuvre)
Coughing, weight lifting, trumpeting, breath-holding attacks

The commonest cause is vaso-vagal syncope (Table 4.1). This has a highly characteristic form. There is usually a precipitating cause or situation. Typical examples include: a frightening, emotional or unpleasant experience or scene, pain, venusection, prolonged standing, and crowded or hot environment. Alcohol or fatigue can predispose to syncope. The syncope is a biphasic reflex. In the first phase, blood pressure begins to drift progressively lower and compensatory measures come into play such as tachycardia and peripheral vascular shutdown (causing pallor). The patient experiences a feeling of light headedness (a feeling of being 'about to faint'), dizziness, nausea, rushing sounds, or greying out of vision (the loss of vision in normal consciousness, which never happens in epilepsy, is due to retinal ischaemia) and sweating may occur. These symptoms can last for several minutes and progressively worsen. The second phase occurs when there is a sudden and massive fall in blood pressure, bradycardia, and peripheral vascodilation. The patient collapses and looses consciousness. There will be pallor, but no cyanosis, and often irregular myoclonic jerking. This phase lasts for a few seconds only (10–30sec usually), and is followed by rapid recovery as the blood pressure is restored, cardiac output increases and cerebral blood flow is resumed. There is no post-ictal confusion or sleep. Incontinence can occur, but is uncommon, and lateral tongue biting is very rare.

In cardiogenic syncope, similar syncopal symptoms occur but without a prodromal phase if cardiac output suddenly ceases (for instance, in cardiac arrhythmia).

Table 4.1 **Differentiating tonic-clonic seizures and vaso-vagal syncope**

Features	Epileptic seizure	Vaso-vagal syncope
Precipitating factor	Uncommon	Very common
Prodromal period	Rare, short	Common, prolonged
Warning	Short stereotyped aura common	Feeling faint, blacking or greying out of vision with preserved consciousness, sweaty, nauseated, panicky, rushing sound in ears
Convulsive movements	Several minutes. Synchronous and rhythmic, initially small amplitude fast evolve to slow large amplitude jerks	Less than 1min, irregular un–coordinated myoclonic jerks
Incontinence	Common	Can occur
Lateral tongue biting	Common	Rare
Injury	Common	Uncommon
Post-ictal	Confusion very common	Rapid recovery without confusion

4.1.2 Psychogenic seizures (syn: dissociative seizures: non-epileptic attack disorder; pseudoseizures)

This condition is, after syncope, the second most commonly mistaken for epilepsy. It tends to occur in patients with a history of abnormal illness behaviour, somatization or with a history of abuse, and is more common in females than males. There is often a psychogenic precipitant. The attacks usually commence in adolescence or early adulthood. The attacks do not occur in sleep or when the patient is alone. The method of description by patients of an attack can be helpful in diagnosis, and patients with psychogenic seizures tend to resist focusing on individual seizure episodes and find it much more difficult to provide a detailed seizure description than patients with epilepsy. A variety of symptoms can occur, but in general, psychogenic seizures tend to take one of the two forms:

- *Motor attacks*. These are superficially like convulsions, although the motor activity is often incoordinated, waxes and wanes, and persists far longer than a convulsion. The rhythmical pattern of a tonic-clonic seizure is not present. There may be distractibility, evidence of awareness, and prominent pelvic movements and back arching (Table 4.2).
- *Motionless attacks*. These attacks take the form of sudden collapse with the patient laying flaccid and motionless, sometimes for many minutes.

4.1.3 Panic attacks and hyperventilation

Panic attacks often include feelings of fear and anxiety, autonomic changes and hyperventilation, dizziness, and light headedness. These can be difficult to differentiate from complex partial seizures, although the psychological context and the situation in which the attacks occur usually aid diagnosis.

Hyperventilation is often associated with panic, but can also occur independently. It produces a characteristic perioral and peripheral tingling sensation (due to altered blood pH) which is not encountered in epilepsy.

4.1.4 Cardiac disorders

Any disorder which lessens cardiac output suddenly carries the risk of reducing cerebral blood flow and causing loss of consciousness. The attacks typically take the form of drop attacks. Arrhythmias are the commonest cardiac disorders entering into the differential diagnosis of epilepsy. These may be acquired, for instance in sick sinus syndrome, or genetic, for instance in long QT syndrome. Mitral valve prolapse, aortic stenosis, and hypertrophic cardiomyopathy also cause blackouts. All patients presenting with apparent epilepsy should be investigated with an electrocardiogram (ECG) and a cardiological opinion sought if there is a possibility of cardiac dysfunction.

Features	Tonic-clonic seizures	Psychogenic seizures (convulsive type)
Table 4.2 Differentiating features of epilepsy and motor psychogenic attacks		
Precipitating cause	Uncommon	In some cases emotion or stress
When alone or asleep	Common	Rare (if at all)
Onset	Rapid	Variable
Aura	Brief, stereotyped	Can be prolonged and variable
Speech during seizure	Cry at onset	Speech can occur
Convulsive movements	Synchronous and rhythmic, initially small amplitude fast evolve to slow large amplitude jerks	Asynchronous flailing of limbs, irregular, wax and wane, pelvic thrusting, opisthotonos
Injury	Lateral tongue biting, accidental injury, posterior dislocation of shoulder, crush vertebral fracture	May bite tongue (usually tip), carpet burns, injury rare; directed violence not uncommon
Consciousness	Complete loss	Variable responsiveness, often possible to communicate
Response to stimulation	None	Often reactive
Incontinence	Common	Sometimes
Duration	Few minutes	Few minutes, may be prolonged

4.1.5 Hypoglycaemia

Hypoglycaemia can cause loss of consciousness. This is most commonly due to insulin therapy in patients with diabetes mellitus or very occasionally because of an insulin secreting tumour. The attacks occur if meals are delayed or missed, there is often a marked prodomal phase of hunger, confusion, anxiety, sweating, fuddled thinking, and unease, symptoms which rapidly resolve with glucose administration. Occasionally there is no prodromal stage. Focal neurological features may occur. Hypoglycaemia should be considered in any patient with prolonged recurrent attacks in which florid or bizarre behaviour is a prominent feature.

4.1.6 Movement disorders and other neurological conditions

Occasionally, movement disorders can be mistaken for epilepsy, including paroxysmal kinesiogenic chorea, tics, bruxism, or paroxysmal dystonia. Patients with learning disability also often have stereotyped or repetitive movements which can be confused with epilepsy and these include stereotypes, head banging, or body rocking.

4.1.7 **Migraine**

The prodrome of migraine can be mistaken for epilepsy, and the differential diagnosis is particularly difficult in relation to visual symptoms which can mimic occipital lobe seizures. However, the tempo is usually different, with migraine gradually evolving over 10–20min, without loss of consciousness. The fortification spectra commonly encountered in migraine do not occur in epilepsy. The prolonged migrainous headache is also a typical feature of migraine, and rare after a simple partial seizure.

4.1.8 **Transient vestibular symptoms**

Acute attacks of dizziness or 'blackout' are common in vestibular disease and can be difficult to distinguish from complex partial seizures, although the dreaminess and perceptual changes do not occur. Other pointers to vestibular disease are deafness, tinnitus, a feeling of pressure in the ear, and relation to head position.

4.1.9 **Episodic phenomena in sleep**

Whole body jerks commonly occur in normal subjects on falling asleep. Fragmentary physiological myoclonus usually involves the peripheries or the face, and occurs during stages 1 and 2 and rapid eye movement (REM) sleep. Periodic movements of sleep are a common phenomenon in older persons, are typically repetitive at regular intervals of 10–60sec and may occur in clusters over many minutes.

4.1.9.1 *Non-REM parasomnias*

These include night terrors or sleep walking. They usually present in childhood or adolescence, and are often familial. The attacks arise from slow-wave sleep, typically at least 30min, but not more than 4hr, after going to sleep. The attacks are usually infrequent, and rarely occur more than once per week and rarely is there more than one attack in a single night. They are exacerbated by stress. In a night terror, there are intense autonomic features (sweating, flushing, palpitations) and a look of fear. Patients may recall a frightening scene or experience, but do not usually recount a vivid dream before the attacks. Vocalization is common. Sleep walking is a curious phenomenon in which complex tasks can be performed without any memory. Speech is usually slow or monosyllabic. Brief, abortive episodes are commoner, involving sitting up in bed with fidgeting and shuffling (mimicking a complex partial seizure).

4.1.9.2 *REM parasomnias*

These events usually occur in middle age or in the elderly, and show a marked male predominance. They more often occur in the later portion of sleep. Attacks may last from seconds to minutes, and take the form of violent movements and vivid 'dreams' that can be partially recalled. Although REM sleep behaviour disorders do occur in healthy elderly subjects they are also seen in association with drugs (e.g. tricyclics) or alcohol, or central nervous system diseases such as multisystem atrophy in which the REM parasomnia can be the presenting symptom.

4.1.10 **Psychiatric symptoms and mental/psychic phenomena**

Transient hallucinatory or affective symptoms are common in many psychiatric conditions, including psychosis, anxiety, depression, and obsessional states. They also occur in such states of sleep deprivation, and can be due to drug ingestion, poisoning, or other toxic states. The context or related symptoms usually make the diagnosis clear, but occasionally the question of epilepsy arises. Recurrent or stereotyped attacks particularly can cause diagnostic confusion with epilepsy. Episodes of déjà vu are frequently experienced by healthy people, but the question of epilepsy sometimes arises. Epileptic déjà vu are usually intense, associated with other features including a dreamy sensation, stereotyped, and have no environmental precipitants. Flashbacks can be due to recreational drug use and also occur in anxiety, depression, and obsessional states.

4.2 **Investigation**

4.2.1 **Electroencephalogram**

This is a functional measure of cerebral activity (Figures 4.1–4.3). A routine interictal EEG is typically recorded for 20–30min, and includes the activation procedures of hyperventilation and photic stimulation. Most EEG departments use 16 channels of EEG arranged according to the International 10–20 system of scalp electrode placement, but additional electrodes are often useful (for instance, sphenoidal electrodes). The role of EEG in epilepsy is summarized in Box 4.3. For diagnostic purposes, it is usual—to perform an EEG in all adults in whom the clinical history suggests an epileptic seizure. In children, EEG is recommended after a second seizure, as the diagnostic yield from routine EEG after a single seizure is considered too low to influence management.

Figure 4.1 Genarialized spike-wave discharge in a patient with IGE manifesting with GTCS on awakening

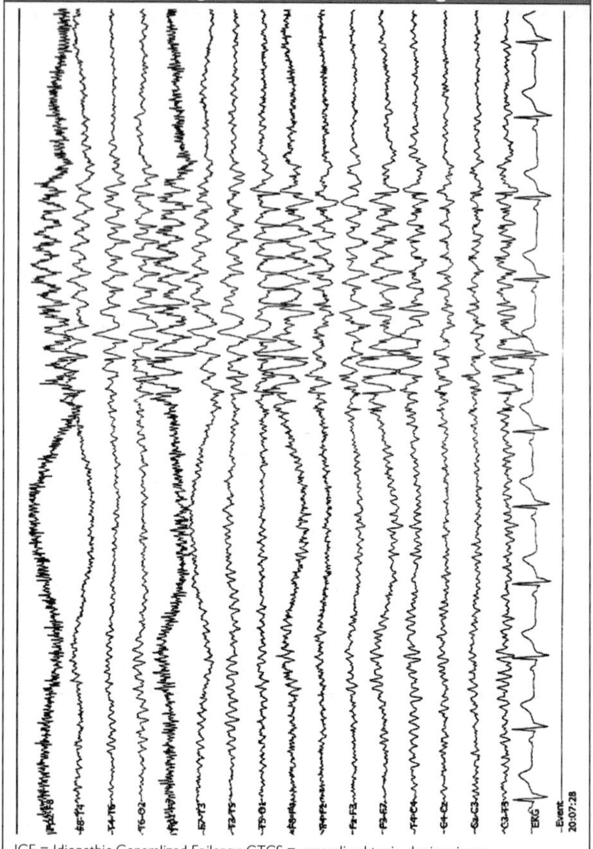

IGE = Idiopathic Generalized Epilepsy; GTCS = generalized tonic-clonic seizure.

Figure 4.2 Ictal EEG: right mesial temporal lobe seizure. Referential recording showing rhythmical 5–7Hz discharge over the right antero-mid temporal lobe

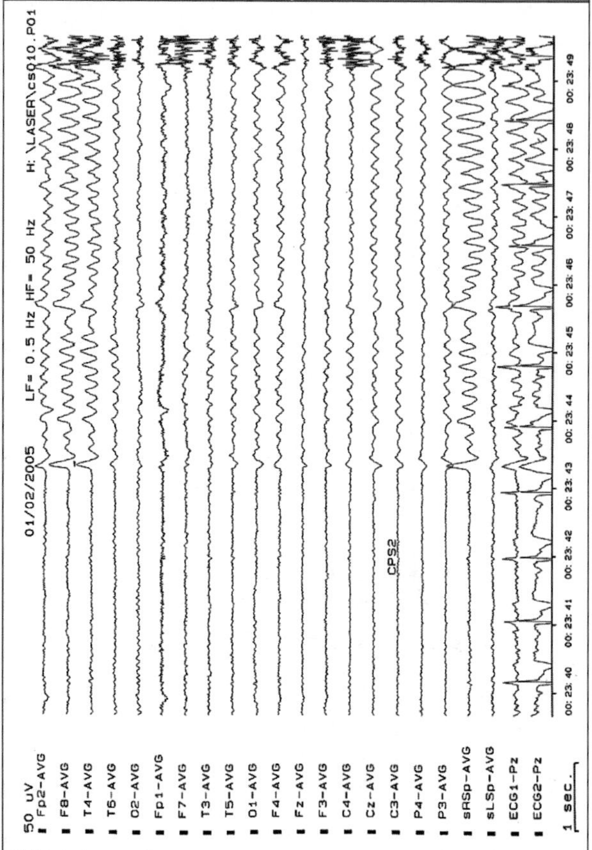

EEG = electroencephalogram.

Figure 4.3 High-frequency interictal discharge in a patient with neocortical or lateral TLE

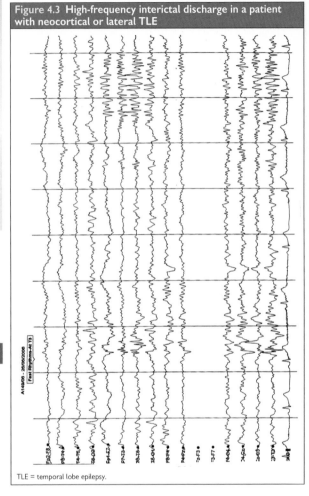

TLE = temporal lobe epilepsy.

EEG interpretation can be complex. The role of interictal EEG in epilepsy is summarized in Box 4.3. It is absolutely vital to provide the reporting neurophysiologist with a clear idea of what question is being asked and to provide sufficient clinical information including details of medication.

Box 4.3 The role of interictal EEG in epilepsy

- To determine whether there are signs of a liability to epilepsy (by the presence of unequivocal epileptiform changes)
- To classify seizures into focal or generalized categories
- To localize and lateralize epileptic foci
- To identify particular changes which aid syndromic classification
- To identify seizure triggers (e.g. photosensitivity)
- To assess the probability of recurrence after a single unprovoked seizure
- To assess the likelihood of seizure recurrence after antiepileptic drug withdrawal in epilepsy in remission
- To assess cognitive dysfunction
- To identify epileptic encephalopathy
- To identify drug side effects

4.2.1.1 *EEG in the diagnosis of epilepsy*

The diagnosis of epilepsy is essentially clinical. However, EEG, if abnormal, is a very useful adjunctive test. It is important to realize though that a normal EEG does not exclude a diagnosis. Up to about half of the patients with epileptic disorders may have one normal interictal EEG, and approximately 10% of patients in routine practice with epilepsy will never show interictal changes. A normal or negative EEG cannot therefore be used to rule out the clinical diagnosis of an epileptic seizure. The specificity of EEG in epilepsy is higher than its sensitivity, but a very small percentage of otherwise normal subjects may show epileptiform abnormalities in their EEG. Epileptiform phenomena may also be seen in 10%–30% of patients who have neurological disorders or cerebral pathologies (e.g. tumour, head injury, cranial surgery), and also in family members in some genetic forms of epilepsy (for instance BECTS) without a history of seizures. EEGs are also very liable to misinterpretation when the reporting physician has insufficient knowledge of the clinical context or question. There are also a range of non-specific EEG phenomena and artefacts that are commonly mistaken for pathological abnormalities. The misinterpretation of EEG, even in experienced hands, is a common reason for a misdiagnosis of epilepsy.

4.2.1.2 *EEG in the classification of epilepsy*

The EEG has an important role in classifying epilepsy into generalized and partial types and in confirming syndromic classifications. For instance, the diagnosis of *Idiopathic Generalized Epilepsy* is strongly supported by the finding of genaralized spike or polyspike and slow-wave discharges at 3–5Hz (see Figure 4.1), normal background cortical

EEG = electroencephalogram.

rhythms, and a relatively high occurrence of photosensitivity. Similarly, the diagnosis of *Lennox–Gastaut Syndrome* is defined by the presence of relatively slow (<2.5Hz) and less regular spike-wave discharge, and the EEG shows abnormalities of background cerebral activity. The EEG is diagnostic of *benign childhood epilepsy with centro-temporal spikes*, the characteristic being high amplitude focal sharp wave discharges in central and temporal regions, either bilateral or unilateral, and potentiated by sleep. Background cerebral rhythms are normal. Focal discharges are helpful in localizing or laterizing an epileptic focus in partial epilepsy (see Figure 4.3), and the EEG is often abnormal even in the presence of infrequent (or indeed any) seizures. Hypsarrhythmia is the diagnostic signature of *West Syndrome* (infantile spasm). Other syndromes also have characteristic EEG findings, particularly in childhood.

The value of EEG can be enhanced by activation procedures, sleep recordings, prolonged EEG recordings (for several hours), ambulatory 24hr recordings (with the patient carrying a recorder, much as the Holter monitoring of the ECG), and in video-EEG telemetry.

Prolonged recordings also have a better chance of recording actual seizures (ictal recordings). Ictal recordings are useful in the differential diagnosis of difficult cases, although this is required in relatively few instances (see Figure 4.2). Ictal recordings are mandatory in pre-surgical assessment. Intracranial EEG is sometimes required, with electrodes placed either on the surface of the brain (grid or strip electrodes) or in the brain substance (depth electrodes).

4.2.1.3 *Other roles for EEG*

The EEG can be useful in determining the cause of cognitive deterioration, either by the identification of subclinical disturbances, encephalopathy, or drug-induced changes.

There is a limited role also for determining prognosis in chronic epilepsy and for estimating the chance of recurrence after a first seizure and after withdrawal of medication in epilepsy in remission. The value of EEG in this situation is greater in the generalized epilepsies, and in particular in Idiopathic Generalized Epilepsy (see Section 2.3.1 and Box 2.8), where the persistence of discrete episodes of spike-wave discharges on a normal background is a significant predictive factor for seizure recurrence.

In the past, EEG was used to detect underlying structural brain disorders, but this role has been completely superceded by neuroimaging with computer tomography (CT) and magnetic resonance imaging (MRI). Similarly, EEG is now seldom used to evaluate psychiatric disorders, a practice which was previously widely employed.

4.2.2 **Magnetic resonance imaging**

MRI is an investigation designed to reveal structure not function—and thus differs importantly in this regard from EEG. Most patients who develop epilepsy or whose chronic epilepsy has not been fully assessed should be investigated with MRI. Although this will depend on availability, in most well-resourced settings, this should be the rule with the only common exception being in patients with unequivocal Idiopathic Generalized Epilepsy.

MRI identifies a causal epileptogenic lesion in approximately 12% of patients with newly diagnosed epilepsy, and in approximately 50% of patients with chronic refractory partial epilepsy (Table 4.3).

The MRI sequences need to be tailored to the clinical question. The primary MRI features of hippocampal sclerosis, for instance, are hippocampal atrophy, demonstrated with coronal T1-weighted images, and increased signal intensity within the hippocampus on T2-weighted images. In addition, decreased T1-weighted signal intensity and disruption of the internal structure of the hippocampus may be present. FLAIR images provide an increased contrast between grey and white matter, and facilitate differentiation of the amygdala from the hippocampus.

4.2.3 Other forms of imaging

Other forms of imaging in epilepsy are of less utility. CT scanning will detect large cortical lesions such as tumour, stroke, trauma but less well than MRI. CT is also helpful in identifying focal cortical calcification and in diagnosing tuberous sclerosis and Sturge–Weber syndrome. However, important pathologies are often invisible on CT, including hippocampal sclerosis, some forms of malformations of cortical development (MCD), small cavernomas, and small lesions in the mesial or basal temporal lobe. CT is required when there are contraindications to MRI, for instance, due to a cardiac pacemaker or cochlear implant. Positron emission tomography (PET) and single photon emission computed tomography (SPECT) scanning have utility in pre-surgical evaluation, but not in most other situations.

Table 4.3 The yield of MRI abnormalities in chronic epilepsy with normal CT	
Abnormality	Yield (%)
None	26
Hippocampal sclerosis	32
Cortical dysgenesis	13
Vascular malformation	8
Tumour	12
Infarct/contusion	6
Other	11

Key: CT = computer tomography; MRI = magnetic resonance imaging.
Note: From a study of 341 patients.

4.2.4 **Electrocardiogram**

As mentioned earlier, all patients with suspected epilepsy should have a routine ECG with measures of the QT interval, to exclude (or at least render unlikely) a primary cardiac cause of blackouts. If there is any suspicion of cardiac dysfunction, referral to a cardiologist is advised.

4.2.5 **Other investigations aimed at determining the cause of epilepsy**

As shown earlier, there are many different causes of epilepsy. Many will be detected by MRI and other imaging technologies, and structural neuro-imaging should be carried out in all patients. All patients with suspected epilepsy should have a full blood count and a full biochemical screen (including measurement of calcium and magnesium levels).

Detailed biochemical examination for inborn errors of metabolism or serological/immunological tests, and other investigations such as a cerebrospinal fluid (CSF) examination, genetic testing, karyotype analysis, or biopsy depend on the clinical circumstances.

References and further reading

Cook M (2009). The differential diagnosis of epilepsy. In SD Shorvon, E Perucca, J Engel, eds. *The treatment of epilepsy*, 3rd edn. Wiley Blackwell, Oxford.

Duncan J, Shorvon S, and Fish D (1995). *Clinical epilepsy*. Churchill Livingstone, New York.

ILAE Commission Report (1997). Recommendations for neuroimaging of patients with epilepsy. Commission on Neuroimaging of the International League Against Epilepsy. *Epilepsia*, **38**, 1255–6.

ILAE Commission Report (1998). Guidelines for neuroimaging evaluation of patients with uncontrolled epilepsy considered for surgery. Commission on Neuroimaging of the International League Against Epilepsy. *Epilepsia*, **39**, 1375–6.

ILAE Commission Report (2000). Commission on Diagnostic Strategies. Recommendations for functional neuroimaging of persons with epilepsy. Neuroimaging Subcommission of the International League Against Epilepsy. *Epilepsia*, **41**, 1350–6.

Koutroumanidis M and Smith SJ (2005). Use and abuse of EEG in the diagnosis of idiopathic generalized epilepsies. *Epilepsia*, **46**, 96–107.

Labar DR (1991). Sleep disorders and epilepsy: differential diagnosis. *Seminars in Neurology*, **11**, 128–34.

Lacey C, Cook MJ, and Salzberg M (2007). The neurologist, psychogenic nonepileptic seizures, and borderline personality disorder. *Epilepsy & Behaviour*, **11**, 492–8.

Leach JP, Stephen LJ, Salveta C, and Brodie MJ (2006). Which EEG for epilepsy? The relative usefulness of different EEG protocols in patients with possible epilepsy. *Journal of Neurology, Neurosurgery, and Psychiatry*, **77**, 1040–2.

Lempert T, Bauer M, and Schmidt D (1994). Syncope: a videometric analysis of 56 episodes of transient cerebral hypoxia. *Annals of Neurology*, **36**, 233–7.

Li LM, Fish DR, Sisodiya SM, Shorvon SD, Alsanjari N, Stevens JM (1995). High resolution magnetic resonance imaging in adults with partial or secondary generalised epilepsy attending a tertiary referral unit. *Journal of Neurology, Neurosurgery, and Psychiatry*, **59**, 384–7.

Mathias CJ and Kimber JR (1999). Postural hypotension: causes, clinical features, investigation, and management. *Annual Review of Medicine*, **50**, 317–36.

Mathias CJ, Deguchi K, and Schatz I (2001). Observations on recurrent syncope and presyncope in 641 patients. *Lancet*, **357**, 348–53.

McGonigal A, Oto M, Russell AJ, Greene J, and Duncan R (2002). Outpatient video EEG recording in the diagnosis of non-epileptic seizures: a randomised controlled trial of simple suggestion techniques. *Journal of Neurology, Neurosurgery, and Psychiatry*; **72**, 549–51.

McKeon A, Vaughan C, and Delanty N (2006). Seizure versus syncope. *Lancet Neurology*, **5**, 171–80.

Meierkord H, Shorvon S, Lightman S, and Trimble M (1992). Comparison of the effects of frontal and temporal lobe partial seizures on prolactin levels. *Archives of Neurology*, **49**, 225–30.

Meierkord H, Will B, Fish D, Shorvon S (1992). The clinical features and prognosis of pseudoseizures diagnosed using video EEG telemetry. *Neurology*, **41**,1643–6.

Montagna P, Lugaresi E, and Plazzi G (1997). Motor disorders in sleep. *European Neurology*, **38**, 190–7.

Muranaka H, Fujita H, Goto A, Osari SI, and Kimura Y (2001). Visual symptoms in epilepsy and migraine: localization and patterns. *Epilepsia*, **42**, 62–6.

Panayiotopoulos CP (1999). Visual phenomena and headache in occipital epilepsy: a review, a systematic study and differentiation from migraine. *Epileptic Disorders*, **1**, 205–16.

Provini F, Plazzi G, and Lugaresi E (Sep 2000). From nocturnal paroxysmal dystonia to nocturnal frontal lobe epilepsy. *Clinical Neurophysiology*, **111**(Suppl 2), S2–8.

Reuber M, Fernandez G, Bauer J, Singh DD, and Elger CE (2002). Interictal EEG abnormalities in patients with psychogenic nonepileptic seizures. *Epilepsia*, **43**, 1013–20.

Riggs JE (2002). Neurologic manifestations of electrolyte disturbances. *Neurologic Clinics*; **20**, 227–39.

Savage DD, Corwin L, McGee DL, Kannel WB, and Wolf PA (1985). Epidemiologic features of isolated syncope: the Framingham Study. *Stroke*, **16**, 626–29.

Shah AK, Shein N, Fuerst D, Yangala R, Shah J, and Watson C (2001). Peripheral WBC count and serum prolactin level in various seizure types and nonepileptic events. *Epilepsia*, **42**, 1472–5.

Chapter 5

Principles of treatment of epilepsy

Key points

- All treatment decisions in epilepsy depend on a balance between the benefits and the drawbacks of therapy, and all treatment decisions should be tailored to the requirements of the individual patient.
- Approximately 70% of people with epilepsy will stop having seizures at some point after the introduction of antiepileptic therapy
- The treatment of newly diagnosed drug-naive epilepsy is more effective than that of chronic epilepsy.
- Treatment protocols should be followed in all situations.
- The choice of antiepileptic drug depends on the type of seizure and on other aspects relating to an individual patient profile.
- The treatment protocols for epilepsy differ in different groups. Some patient groups have specific issues, for instance, children, the elderly, those with learning disability, and women of child-bearing age.

5.1 Principles of treatment of newly diagnosed or drug-naive patients

All treatment decisions in epilepsy depend on a balance between the benefits and the drawbacks of therapy, and all treatment decisions should be tailored to the requirements of the individual patient. These guiding principles apply to all clinical situations, but are particularly relevant when it comes to deciding whether to initiate treatment in newly diagnosed, drug-naive patients. The balance can be difficult to decide. The benefits of therapy include the lower risk of recurrence of seizures, and thus of potential injury and even death, and the psychological and social benefits of more security from seizures. The drawbacks of therapy include the potential drug side effects, the psychological and social effects of 'being epileptic', the cost, and inconvenience.

The factors that influence the decision are as follows:

5.1.1 Diagnosis

It is essential to establish a firm diagnosis of epilepsy before therapy is started. There is almost no place at all for a 'trial of treatment' to clarify the diagnosis, as it seldom does. Follow-up may be necessary before a diagnosis becomes clarified, and indeed it may take months or years before a diagnosis is achieved with certainty. It is in general terms still better to withhold rather than initiate therapy in cases of uncertainty, in spite of the length of observation that might be necessary.

5.1.2 Risk of recurrence of seizure

The estimation of risk of seizure recurrence is obviously a key factor in deciding whether to initiate therapy. Over 50% of all patients who have a first non-febrile seizure will have further attacks. The risk of recurrence is high initially (44% in the 6 months after the first seizure) and then progressively falls (32% in the next 6 months and 17% in the second year) (Figure 5.1). If two or more spontaneous seizures have occurred, the risk of further attacks in the future without treatment is, in most clinical circumstances, over 80%. Aetiology is an important predictor of recurrence risk. The risk is higher in those with structural cerebral disease, and least in acute symptomatic seizures provoked by metabolic or drug and/or toxin exposure (Figure 5.2). The risk of recurrence of 'idiopathic' or 'cryptogenic' seizures is approximately 50%. Electroencephalogram (EEG) changes have some utility in predicting recurrence. If the EEG shows spike and wave discharges, the risk of recurrence is higher. Other changes have less predictive value. The predictive value of an EEG showing other abnormalities after a single seizure, such as focal slowing, is slight. A normal EEG has also little predictive value. Age is relevant and the risk of recurrence is somewhat greater in those under the age of 16 or over the age of 60yrs. Seizure type and syndrome are also important predictors of recurrence.

5.1.3 Type, timing, and frequency of the seizures

Some types of epileptic seizure have a minimal impact on the quality of life; for example, simple partial seizures, absence, or sleep attacks. The benefits of treating such seizures, even if happening frequently, can be outweighed by the disadvantages. Similarly, if the baseline seizure frequency is very low, even if the seizures take a severe form, the disadvantages of treatment can be unacceptably high. However, tonic-clonic seizures carry a risk of accidents or even death, and treatment is commonly recommended after an isolated first tonic-clonic seizure.

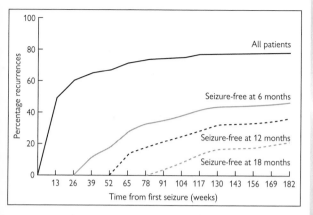

Figure 5.1 This figure shows the risk of recurrence of seizures after a first attack in a population-based prospective study of 564 patients with new-onset seizures: for all patients and for those who had had a recurrence at 6, 12, and 18 months after the first attack (figures from the National General Practice Study of Epilepsy).

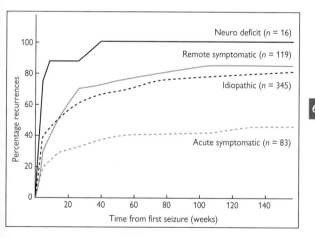

Figure 5.2 This figure shows the risk of recurrence after a first seizure in different epilepsy categories from the same study of 564 patients with new-onset seizures (figures from the National General Practice Study of Epilepsy).

5.1.4 **Treatment protocol for initial treatment**

All patients with new-onset seizures should be referred for specialist advice, in order to establish diagnosis and choose appropriate treatment regimens. The principles of therapy in newly diagnosed epilepsy are summarized in Box 5.1.

5.1.4.1 *Establish diagnosis*

Almost all patients will require EEG and neuroimaging, and other investigations as necessary. Neuroimaging should be with magnetic resonance imaging (MRI) scanning in all patients with partial-onset epilepsy or epilepsy developing after the age of 15 without good explanation. The MRI must be of high quality, of 1.5 or 3 Tesla, with T1-, T2-weighted, and fluid attenuated inversion recovery (FLAIR) sequences, and preferably with a thin slice volume acquisition that allows further reformatting and quantification.

5.1.4.2 *Identify and counsel about precipitating factors*

If precipitating factors can be avoided, this occasionally obviates the need for drug therapy altogether. Even if drug treatment is needed, advice about lifestyle and avoiding precipitating factors is essential and can greatly improve the response to therapy.

5.1.4.3 *Decide upon the need for antiepileptic drug therapy*

If therapy is needed, baseline biochemical and haematological parameters should be measured.

Box 5.1 Principles of treatment of newly diagnosed patients

- Aim for complete control without adverse effects
- Diagnosis of epileptic seizures should be unequivocal
- Seizure type, syndrome, and aetiology should be established
- Baseline haematological and biochemical investigations should be performed before drug initiation
- Therapy should be started using a single drug (monotherapy)
- Initial titration should be to low-maintenance doses
- Further upward titration will depend on response and side effects
- If first drug fails, alternative monotherapies should be tried
- Upward and downward titration should be in slow stepped doses
- Polytherapy should be used only if monotherapy with at least three first-choice drugs has failed to control seizures
- Patients should be fully counselled about goals, role, risk, outcome, and logistics of drug treatment

5.1.4.4 *Advise about the goals, likely outcome, risks, and logistics of therapy*

This advice should include an appropriate warning of potential side effects should be given. Some drugs carry a risk of idiosyncratic reactions, and patients should be instructed to seek immediate medical attention if signs of hypersensitivity or idiosyncratic drug reactions develop.

5.1.4.5 *Drug therapy*

A suitable drug should be chosen—see section 5.3. This should be started in monotherapy, initially at low doses, and titrated up slowly to a low-maintenance dose. Drug loading at high doses is not necessary except in emergencies.

If seizures continue: the drug dosage should be titrated upwards to higher maintenance dose levels (guided, where appropriate, by serum level monitoring). In approximately 60%–70% of patients, these simple steps for initial therapy will result in complete seizure control.

If seizures still continue: despite good doses of the initial monotherapy, an alternative monotherapy should be tried with another appropriate first-choice antiepileptic drug. The second drug should be introduced incrementally at suitable dose intervals, and the first drug then withdrawn in slow decremental steps. The second drug should be titrated first to low-maintenance doses, and if seizures continue, the dose increased incrementally to maximal doses. If seizures still continue, a third alternative monotherapy should be tried in the same manner.

If seizures persist, at any time during this process, the diagnosis should be reassessed, and in this situation it is not uncommon to find that the attacks do not have an epileptic basis. Investigation should also be considered to exclude the possibility of a progressive lesion. The possibility of poor compliance should be explored.

5.2 Treatment of patients with chronic active epilepsy

Chronic epilepsy can be defined as *epilepsy in which seizures are still occurring 5 or more years after the initiation of therapy*. Chronic epilepsy is more difficult to treat than newly diagnosed epilepsy, and this curious fact has interested researchers for several decades. The reasons are not clear, but there are two possible hypotheses. It is possible that the longer epilepsy remains active, the more resistant it becomes to treatment, perhaps because of the many molecular changes that occur in ongoing epilepsy (in other words, as famously noted by Sir William Gowers in 1888, 'seizures beget seizures'). Alternatively, it is possible that chronic epilepsy comprises the inherently more severe forms of the condition that were unresponsive to therapy from the very start of therapy (i.e. at the time of diagnosis and first treatment), and that the higher frequency of resistant cases in chronic epilepsy reflects simply the fact that the easier to treat responsive cases are selected out early in the course of the condition. Whatever the explanation, repeated studies have demonstrated that (a) in approximately 60%–70% of patients with newly diagnosed epilepsy, seizures will cease within the first months or few years of therapy, and the epilepsy will enter long-term remission; and (b) that the rate of long-term remission in chronic epilepsy is much lower. It is possible though that the prognosis has improved over recent years because of the much wider range of medication that is now available.

When first seeing a patient with chronic uncontrolled epilepsy, a two-stage procedure should be adopted. First, an assessment of diagnosis and previous treatment history should be made. As a second step, a treatment plan should be devised.

5.2.1 Assessment

5.2.1.1 *Review the diagnosis of epilepsy*

It may be surprising to know that 20% or more of patients referred to neurology clinics with chronic epilepsy do not in fact suffer from epilepsy at all. Many different conditions may be confused with epilepsy, but the commonest are psychogenic seizures, reflex syncope, and cardiac arrhythmia. An eye witnessed account of the attacks should be obtained and will usually be diagnostic. A series of normal EEG results should alert one to the possibility that the attacks are non-epileptic, although this is not an infallible rule. An invaluable aid to diagnosis can be the viewing of a recording of the attack made by home video or on a mobile phone.

5.2.1.2 *Establish aetiology*

The cause of the epilepsy must be established. This is important as specific cerebral conditions may require therapy in their own right, and also because prognosis and response to therapy are strongly influenced by the underlying cause. This may require MRI scanning and/or other investigations. A high-quality MRI scan is a mandatory test in a patient with chronic epilepsy without a known cause.

5.2.1.3 *Classify seizure type and syndrome*

This guides the choice of medication (see section 5.3 Drug choice). Accurate seizure and syndrome classification requires a detailed clinical history and EEG.

5.2.1.4 *Review previous treatment history*

The response to an antiepileptic drug is, generally speaking, relatively consistent over time. A knowledge of the previous treatment history is vital to the formulation of a rational treatment plan. Poor compliance can be a reason for poor seizure control.

5.2.2 **Treatment plan (a series of treatment trials)**

A key step in the successful treatment of chronic epilepsy is the development of a treatment plan. This should be based on the assessment, and the plan should be documented in medical records and discussed with the patient.

Although, meta-analysis has shown that none of the currently available first- and second-line drugs is significantly better than any other in population terms, one thing is clear—that individual patients who have failed to respond to one drug may well respond to an alternative. It follows from this that the only logical approach to antiepileptic drug treatment, in a patient in whom improvement in seizure control is desired, is to try one suitable drug after another. The treatment plan therefore should comprise, at its heart, a sequence of what are in effect $n = 1$ treatment trials, each to be tried in turn if the previous trial fails to meet the targeted level of seizure control.

The effectiveness of this approach was shown in one study in which a total of 265 drug additions were studied in 155 adult patients with chronic epilepsy (defined as epilepsy active at least 5yrs after and initiation of therapy). Other therapy was varied (and some drugs withdrawn) according to normal clinic practice. If one drug addition was ineffective, another would be tried. Of the 155 patients, the study found that after one, two, or three drug additions, 28% overall were rendered seizure free by this protocol of active medication change. Sixteen per cent of all drug additions resulted in seizure freedom (defined as seizure freedom at last follow-up for 12 months or longer), and a 50%–99% seizure reduction occurred in a further 21%.

Such a sequence of drug changes can take months to complete and requires patience and tenacity. The procedure should be explained in advance to the patient to maintain confidence and compliance. Ideally, each antiepileptic should be tried in a reasonable dose added to a baseline drug regimen—usually one or two other antiepileptic drugs—and as the drug is added, withdrawal or change in dose of other drugs may be needed. Thus decisions have to be made about (a) which drugs to trial and in what sequence, and which drugs to retain as a baseline regimen; (b) which drugs to withdraw; and (c) the duration of each treatment trial.

5.2.2.1 *Choice of drug to trial and to retain as the baseline regimen*
The drugs should be selected from those that have either not been previously used in optimal doses or those that have been used and did prove helpful. Rational choices therefore depend on a well-documented history of previous drug therapy. The choice of drug also will depend on seizure type, side effects, interactions, the patient profile, personal preference, and other factors—and these are outlined further in section 5.3.

The new drugs added to a regimen should be introduced slowly. This results in better tolerability. It is usual to aim initially for a low-maintenance dose and then to titrate upwards depending on response, but in severe epilepsy, higher doses are often required right away.

5.2.2.2 *Choice of drugs to withdraw and the drug withdrawal process*

Drugs that should be considered for withdrawal are those that have been given in the past in an adequate trial at optimal doses and those that were either ineffective or caused unacceptable side effects. Drug withdrawal needs care, and should be carried out in a gradual step-wise fashion. The sudden reduction in dose of an antiepileptic drug can result in a severe worsening of seizures or in status epilepticus. Only one drug should be withdrawn at a time. If the withdrawal period is likely to be difficult, the dangers can be reduced by covering withdrawal with a benzodiazepine drug (usually clobazam 10mg once a day), given during the phase of active withdrawal. A benzodiazepine can also be given in clustering of seizures following withdrawal. If seizures dramatically worsen during the period of withdrawal, the drug should usually be rapidly reinstated. The patient should have access to immediate specialist advice during a withdrawal period.

5.2.2.3 *Duration of treatment trial*

This will depend on the baseline seizure rate and patterns. The trial should be long enough to have differentiated the effect of therapy from that of chance fluctuations in seizures.

5.2.2.4 *Intractability and the limits of drug therapy*

Drug therapy will fail to control seizures completely in approximately 10%–20% of patients with epilepsy. In this situation, the epilepsy can be categorized as 'intractable' and therapy should provide in these patients the best compromise between inadequate seizure control and drug-induced side effects. Individual patients will take very different view about where to strike this balance. Intractability is inevitably an arbitrary decision.

5.2.2.5 *Serum level monitoring and drug interactions*

For drugs where effectiveness and/or side effects are closely linked to serum level—notably phenytoin, carbamazepine, and phenobarbital—measurement of the serum level can be helpful in deciding dosage. Monitoring serum level is particularly important for phenytoin that has a non-linear relationship between dose and serum level. Drug interactions are another important aspect of therapy with antiepileptic drugs. The usual indications for serum level monitoring are shown in Box 5.2.

Box 5.2 Usual indications for serum level monitoring

- To assess blood levels where there is a poor therapeutic response in spite of adequate dosage
- To identify the cause of adverse effects where these might be drug induced
- To measure pharmacokinetic changes in the presence of physiological or pathological conditions known to alter drug disposition (e.g. pregnancy, liver disease, renal failure, gastrointestinal disease, hypoalbulinaemic states)
- To identify and minimize the consequence of adverse drug interactions in patients receiving multiple-drug therapy
- To monitor dose requirements in drugs with non-linear dose/serum level curves (especially phenytoin)
- To identify poor compliance

5.3 Drug choice

The choice of drug is one of the most important decisions to make—both in patients with newly diagnosed epilepsy and in those with chronic epilepsy. Advice in this area requires experience, and it is in this area particularly that a specialist referral is worthwhile.

In newly diagnosed epilepsy, the range of suitable first-line drugs, licensed for monotherapy in drug-naive patients is more restricted than the choice in chronic epilepsy. Seizure type is an important consideration and the usual drugs given as first-line therapy are shown in Table 5.1. Of these, carbamazepine is the most common first-line drug for partial epilepsy and valproate for generalized epilepsy and especially in *Idiopathic Generalized Epilepsy*.

In chronic epilepsy, drug choice is wider—and the drugs for specific seizure types are shown in Table 5.2. It must be stressed, however, that seizure type is not the only factor to consider in choosing a suitable antiepileptic drug in chronic epilepsy. The patient profile, the nature of potential side effects, the risk of drug interactions, and the balance between side effects and effectiveness are also important (Box 5.3).

The decision about treatment must be made ultimately by the patient, and the role of the doctor is to assess the patient profile and requirements and provide advice and what is in essence is an option appraisal. People differ in their willingness to risk adverse effects, or to try new therapy, and the decision must be made in partnership with the patient and with fully informed consent.

Table 5.1 Newly diagnosed patients: choice of initial monotherapy

Seizure type	Drug
Partial seizures, secondarily generalized tonic-clonic seizures, primary generalized tonic-clonic seizures	Carbamazepine, lamotrigine, levetiracetam, oxcarbazepine, valproate
Absence seizures (typical absence)	Lamotrigine, levetiracetam, valproate
Myoclonic seizures	Levetiracetam, valproate
Atypical absence, tonic and atonic seizures	Lamotrigine, levetiracetam, topiramate, valproate

Table 5.2 Choice of medication in different seizure types in chronic epilepsy

Seizure type	Drugs that show efficacy	Drugs that may worsen seizures
Partial seizures, secondarily generalized tonic-clonic seizures, primary generalized tonic-clonic seizures	Acetazolamide, clobazam, clonazepam, carbamazepine, felbamate, gabapentin, lamotrigine, lacosamide, levetiracetam, oxcarbazepine, phenobarbital, phenytoin, pregabalin, primidone, tiagabine, topiramate, valproate, vigabatrin, zonisamide	
Absence seizures (typical absence)	Acetazolamide, clobazam, clonazepam, ethosuximide, lamotrigine, levetiracetam, phenobarbital, topiramate, valproate	Carbamazepine, gabapentin, oxcarbazepine, tiagabine, vigabatrin
Myoclonic seizures	Clobazam, clonazepam, lamotrigine, levetiracetam, phenobarbital, piracetam, topiramate, valproate	Carbamazepine, gabapentin, oxcarbazepine, phenytoin, tiagabine, vigabatrin
Atypical absence, tonic and atonic seizures	Acetazolamide, clobazam, clonazepam, lamotrigine, levetiracetam, phenobarbital, phenytoin, primidone, topiramate, valproate, zonisamide	Carbamazepine, gabapentin, oxcarbazepine, phenytoin, tiagabine, vigabatrin

74

5.3.1 Side effects

Amongst the most important side effects to consider are the effects on (a) weight—and those who are overweight might be keener to try topiramate or zonisamide, which both typically result in weight loss, rather than gabapentin, pregabalin, or valproate, which typically

Box 5.3 Factors influencing choice of treatment regimen in epilepsy

Personal, patient-related factors

Age and gender

Physical co-morbidity

Emotional, personality, and affective status

Psychiatric co-morbidity

Attitude to risks of seizures and of medication

Social circumstances (employment, education, domestic, etc.)

Factors related to the drug

Mechanism of action

Strength of therapeutic effects

Strength and nature of side effects

Formulation

Drug interactions and pharmacokinetic properties

Cost

The importance of these factors will vary from individual to individual. Interestingly, aetiology is generally not a factor dictating choice of treatment.

---

result in weight gain. (b) Psychological effects—the patient's affective and psychological states are important considerations in drug choice. Some drugs, notably valproate and carbamazepine, tend to stabilize mood. Levetiracetam tends to cause anxiety and agitation, and occasionally more severe behavioural or psychiatric changes, particularly so in patients already anxious or agitated. Phenobarbital and the benzodiazepines tend to exacerbate depression and sedation. (c) Teratogenicity—in women planning to embark on pregnancy, valproate is relatively contraindicated and only carbamazepine and lamotrigine have proven relative safety. (d) Cosmetic effects—phenytoin and barbiturate are associated with long-term cosmetic effects not shared with other antiepileptics. Valproate can cause hair loss. (e) Cognitive impairment—some drugs, notably topiramate, zonisamide, and phenobarbital have reputations for being more likely to result in sedation or cognitive impairment than other drugs.

5.3.2 Drug interactions

These are important considerations in other patients on complex medication regimens. Interactions with antibiotics, anti-neoplastic agents, steroids, warfarin, immunological agents, drugs used in transplantation, and other antiepileptic drugs can be very marked and the co-prescription of an enzyme-inducing antiepileptic drug may seriously impair the efficacy of the other compound. Carbamazepine, phenytoin, phenobarbital, primidone, tiagabine, and valproate are particularly problematic in this regard, whereas gabapentin, and vigabatrin have few interactions, and pregabalin none at all.

5.3.3 **Other factors**

Various other factors are also important. Some patients' preferences depend on aspects such as age, gender, co-morbidity, co-medication, drug formulation and dosing frequencies, and a range of social aspects. Cost is also a consideration in some health-care settings.

5.4 **Treatment of patients with epilepsy in remission**

Epilepsy can be said to be in remission when seizures have not occurred over long time periods (conventionally 2 or 5yrs). Remission occurs, at some point after diagnosis, in some 70%–80% of patients who are diagnosed as having epilepsy. The clinical management of patients in remission is usefully straightforward. Drug doses should be minimized, and it is usually possible to avoid major adverse effects. The seizure type, epilepsy syndrome, aetiology, investigations, and previous treatment should be recorded. Routine haematological or biochemical checks are recommended on an annual basis in an asymptomatic individual. The risk of long-term side effects (e.g. bone disease in post-menopausal women) should be assessed periodically, and the patient should be counselled about issues such as pregnancy where appropriate. In most cases, little medical input is required with appropriate care provided at primary care level and annual visits to the specialist. The question of discontinuing drug therapy also often arises.

5.4.1 **Discontinuation of drug therapy in patients in seizure-remission**

It is often difficult to decide when (if ever) to discontinue drug treatment. The decision should be made by a specialist who is able to provide an estimate of the risk of reactivation of the epilepsy. This risk is influenced by the factors listed below but it must be stressed to all patients that (a) drug withdrawal is never entirely risk free and that in some patients seizures will recur; and furthermore (b) that if seizures do recur, it may be difficult to re-establish full seizure control even if drugs are reinstated (this seems to be the case in approximately 10% of patients in whom seizures recur after drugs are withdrawn). The decision about whether to withdraw therapy will depend on *the level of risk* the patient is prepared to accept.

The best estimates for the probability of remaining seizure free after drug withdrawal come from the Medical Research Council (MRC) Antiepileptic Drug Withdrawal Study, which included 1,013 patients who had been seizure free for 2yrs or more and were randomized to drug withdrawal or continuation of therapy. Within 2 years of starting drug withdrawal 59% remained seizure free compared to 79% of those who were randomized to continuing therapy.

Various factors influence the probability of remaining seizure free:

- *Seizure-free period*: the longer the patient is seizure free, the less likely is the chance of relapse. The overall risk of relapse after drug withdrawal, for instance, after a 5yr seizure-free period is approximately 10%.
- *Duration of active epilepsy*: The longer the history of active seizures (i.e. the duration of time from the onset of epilepsy to the onset of remission), the greater the risk of relapse.
- *Type and severity of epilepsy*: The type of epilepsy and its aetiology are important influences on prognosis. The presence of symptomatic epilepsy, secondarily generalized or myoclonic seizures, neurological deficit, or learning disability greatly lessen the chance of remission, and also increase the chances of recurrence should remission occur. The higher the number of seizures before remission, the greater the number of drugs being taken to control the seizures and the presence of two or more seizure types (a surrogate for severity of epilepsy) all increase the risk of relapse.
- *EEG*: The persistence of spike-wave in those with Idiopathic Generalized Epilepsy is the most useful prognostic EEG feature, indicating a higher chance of relapse. Other EEG abnormalities have no great prognostic utility, and the presence of focal spikes or changes to EEG background in adults are of little help in estimating the chances of remission or relapse after drug withdrawal.

5.4.2 **How to withdraw therapy—the importance of slow reduction**

When a decision to withdraw therapy is made, the drugs should be discontinued in a slow step-wise fashion, which typically takes months to achieve. Fifty per cent of patients who are going to experience seizure recurrence on withdrawal do so during the reduction phase, and 25% in the first 6 months after withdrawal; this should be explained carefully to the patient, and driving restrictions should be applied during the withdrawal period and the subsequent months. In general terms, the slower the withdrawal, the less likely are seizures to recur. The typical rates of reduction of individual drugs are shown in Table 5.3.

If seizures do recur, the drug should be immediately restarted at the dosage that controlled the attacks. Approximately 10% of patients will not regain full remission even if the drug is replaced at the dosage that previously resulted in long remission. Why this should be the case is unclear, but in some patients at least, it seems that recurrence alters subsequent seizure risk.

Table 5.3 Typical rates of withdrawal of antiepileptic drugs

Drug	Step-wise dose decrements (mg) per month
Carbamazepine	100–200
Clobazam	10
Clonazepam	0.25
Ethosuximide	250
Gabapentin	300–400
Lamotrigine	50–100
Levetiracetam	250–500
Oxcarbazepine	150–300
Phenobarbital	15–30
Phenytoin	50–100
Pregabalin	50
Primidone	125–250
Tiagabine	4–5
Topiramate	25
Valproate	200–500
Vigabatrin	500
Zonisamide	50

A range is sometimes given. At higher doses, the higher decremental dose reductions can be usually made, and at the lowest doses the smaller decremental steps.

5.5 Epilepsy in people with learning disability

People with learning disabilities are 30 times more likely to have epilepsy than those without learning disabilities. The risk of epilepsy is over 50% in those with severe learning disabilities and additional motor and sensory impairments. Although the management of epilepsy follows the same general lines as in people without learning disability, there are some specific problems that are important to recognize:

5.5.1 Assessment

The evaluation of epilepsy in people with learning disabilities is compounded by difficulties with communication, co-existence of mental illness, and by other symptoms mimicking epileptic seizures. The history may be less easy to obtain because of poorer adaptive and social skills and additional speech difficulties. It is common to make a diagnosis and decisions about treatment based on carers' reports, and not the history from the individual ('management by proxy').

This is not always satisfactory and the physician should be aware of the lack of reliability of such reports. It is important to keep the primary focus on the needs of the individual patient.

Diagnosis may be more difficult, not only because of difficulties in obtaining an accurate history, but also because epileptic seizures can take unusual forms. Furthermore, there are various motor or behavioural phenomena that occur in people with learning disability, such as mannerisms or stereotyped movements, which are sometimes difficult to differentiate from epileptic seizures. Challenging behaviour, episodic rage, or aggression are sometimes attributed to seizures, although in fact it is rare for epilepsy to directly cause these symptoms, and this misattribution results commonly in inappropriate treatment. There is furthermore a rather nihilistic tendency to underinvestigate epilepsy, which should be resisted.

People with learning disability and epilepsy are twice as likely as others to experience affective disorder and other mental-health problems. The symptoms of depression are often attributed to the learning disability and overlooked ('diagnostic overshadowing'). It is important to be aware of this, and also to survey other factors potentially implicated in behavioural change such as antiepileptic drug intoxication. Non-epileptic attack disorders are more common in people with learning disability who have limited communication skills to express emotional conflicts.

5.5.2 Treatment

As for all those with epilepsy, antiepileptic medication constitutes the first-line of treatment. However, seizures remain poorly controlled in approximately 68% of persons with learning disabilities, despite the fact that 40% or more regularly take more than one antiepileptic drug.

The type of epilepsy also influences response to therapy, but even in severe epilepsy syndromes, an active approach to therapy will often improve seizure control, and the skilful use of appropriate medication can be very beneficial. For instance, in the Lennox–Gastaut syndrome, open non-randomized studies have shown 50% or greater reductions in seizures in between 33% and 74% in patients treated with lamotrigine, vigabatrin, rufinamide, or topiramate.

Seizure reduction should not be the only parameter to consider. Broader quality of life issues are important. The UK government 2001 White Paper emphasizes the need to involve the person with learning disabilities and to devise individually planned care. This is an important principle, and it is essential to consider an individual's own concerns that sometimes revolve much more around issues of side effects or behaviour than seizures.

5.6 **Epilepsy in the elderly**

Approximately 30% of new cases now occur in people over 65yrs, and currently, approximately 0.7% of the elderly population are treated for epilepsy, making epilepsy the third most common serious neurological condition in the elderly after dementia and stroke. As the number of elderly people in the population is rising, the numbers of elderly people requiring treatment for epilepsy is also greatly increasing.

5.6.1 **Causes and diagnosis**

The chief cause of epilepsy in those over 65yrs is cerebrovascular disease. However, tumours and degenerative diseases (including dementia) can present with epilepsy and the cause of seizures should be as actively sought as in younger patients. Diagnosis is not always easy, and care must be made to differentiate epilepsy from cardiac arrhythmia, syncope, vascular disease, transient global amnesia, vertigo, and non-specific 'funny turns'. The greatest difficulty resides in the differentiation from syncope including cardiac syncope, and diagnosis may be complicated by co-morbidity.

Misdiagnosis of epilepsy is common in this age group, and can have serious consequences.

5.6.2 **General aspects of management**

The diagnosis of epilepsy in an elderly person can mark a watershed in that person's life. The experience may seem a harbinger of death, the diagnosis can affect the attitude of others, and may lead to marginalization and disempowerment. It may result in a transition from independent living to the transfer into care. There is a strong tendency to over-react. Management should involve doctors and other professionals, who should maintain as far as possible a synoptical perspective. Confidence needs to be rebuilt; mobility restored; the home circumstances reviewed; and input from social services, remedial, and occupational therapists is often needed. A personal alarm can be very useful, as can counselling and written advice for friends and relatives. Uncontrolled seizures are likely to be more hazardous in an elderly patient. Convulsive attacks carry greater risks in patients with cardiorespiratory disorders, and the old, fragile patient would be more susceptible to suffer from fractures as a consequence of seizures and falls. Compliance with medication can be compromised by memory lapses, failing intellect, or confusion. In these situations, drug administration should be supervised.

5.6.3 **Pharmacokinetic differences**

The relationship between dose and serum level is more variable in the elderly than in young adults. Published pharmacokinetic values are often expressed as mean values that do not necessarily take into account this wider range. Protein binding may be reduced as albumin concentrations are lower, clearance is often lower due to reduced renal function, and the volume of distribution for lipid soluble drugs is often increased. For all these reasons, the half-life of many drugs is longer than in young adults.

5.6.4 **Drug interactions**

Drug interactions are common. In the United States, people over the age of 65 comprise 13% of the population yet receive 32% of pre-scribed medications. In one study of epilepsy patients over 65yrs of age, a mean of 5.6 medications (antiepileptic and non–antiepileptic) per patient was taken.

5.6.5 **Pharmacodynamic differences and side effects**

The elderly are more sensitive to the neurological side effects of drugs, and lower drug doses are sufficient to control seizures in the elderly compared to younger adults. The adverse effects of drugs in the elderly may take unfamiliar forms. Confusion, general ill health, affective change, or uncharacteristic motor or behavioural distur-bances can occur with many antiepileptic drugs. For these reasons, the 'therapeutic ranges' defined in younger age groups should be generally adjusted downwards. Vigilance for unusual side effects should be maintained—both neurological and also metabolic.

Membrane-stabilizing drugs (e.g. phenytoin, carbamazepine, lamo-trigine) carry a higher risk in the elderly of promoting cardiac arrhythmia and hypotension. The enzyme-inducing drugs may increase the propensity to develop osteopenia or osteoporosis. Phenytoin and carbamazepine also pose potential threat and should be used cautiously in individuals with autonomic dysfunction, for instance, in diabetes. Carbamazepine has an antimuscarinic effect that can pre-cipitate urinary retention.

5.6.6 **Drug dosing and regimens**

For all the aforementioned reasons, therapy should generally be initiated with lower doses than in the young adult. Renal and hepatic function and plasma protein concentrations should be measured before therapy is started. Blood level measurements should be made at regular interval, for relevant drugs, at least until stable regimens have been achieved. Drug combinations should be avoided where possible, and the advantages of monotherapy over polytherapy are greater in the elderly than in young adults. Co-morbidity is also very common and this may well affect the choice of medication, not least intercurrent cerebral, hepatic, or renal disease. Many of the drugs given to elderly patients are used in lower dosages than in the for-mularies because renal or hepatic impairment and other co-morbidities are relatively common and a cautious approach to pre-scribina is therefore recommended.

5.6.7 **Individual drugs**

Most drugs have not been subjected to rigorous trials in the elderly, and as a result, data on the use of antiepileptic drugs in the elderly is generally sparse. More studies in this area are urgently required.

5.6.7.1 *Carbamazepine*

Carbamazepine is often used as first-line therapy in partial seizures. However, the pharmacokinetics of carbamazepine are altered by age often in an unpredictable manner and side effects are common. Hyponatraemia can be troublesome and there is a small risk of drug-induced osteoporosis. Elderly patients are more vulnerable to drug-induced impairment of gait, as well as action and postural tremor, and possibly other subtle adverse neurological effects. The drug should be initiated slowly, the modified release formulation should always be used, and maintenance dose should be generally lower (400mg/day is a common initial target dose).

5.6.7.2 *Gabapentin*

Gabapentin is not metabolized and there is minimal protein binding, age-related changes in distribution. These are clear advantages for use in the elderly particularly; however, the age-related changes in renal function in the elderly significantly reduce the renal clearance of gabapentin and thus the dose should be reduced in the elderly, if renal function is impaired.

5.6.7.3 *Lamotrigine*

Lamotrigine has been shown to be effective and well tolerated in elderly patients, and is now often preferred over carbamazepine. There are, however, pharmacokinetic differences in the disposition of lamotrigine in the elderly and the plasma clearance of lamotrigine is reduced by approximately one-third when compared to young adults. The drug is approximately 55% bound to plasma proteins and undergoes extensive hepatic metabolism, and also interacts with other antiepileptic drugs. It is wise to initiate therapy at lower doses in young adults. Recommended maintenance doses are 100mg in monotherapy, 50–100mg when co-medicated with valproate alone, or 200mg in patients co-medicated with other enzyme-inducing antiepileptic drugs.

5.6.7.4 *Levetiracetam*

This drug has few drug interactions and simple pharmacokinetics, which are advantages in the elderly, and recent studies have shown good efficacy and safety. Age-related changes in renal function can affect the clearance of the drug, and doses should be accordingly reduced. An initial dose of 125–250mg is recommended, with incremental steps of 125–250mg until an initial maintenance dose of 750–1,500mg/day is reached.

5.6.7.5 *Phenobarbital*

Phenobarbital was widely used in the elderly, but in recent years it has fallen from fashion because of the risk of neurological and psychiatric side effects. The elderly seem more sensitive to the sedative side effects of phenobarbital, especially when co-medicated with benzodiazepine. The usual starting dose is 30–60mg at night, and dose increments should be cautious and carefully monitored.

5.6.7.6 *Phenytoin*

The pharmacokinetics of phenytoin make it a generally unsuitable drug in the elderly, but it is nevertheless commonly prescribed. It would be wise to initiate therapy at a relatively low dose (initial maintenance dose of 200mg/day) and measurements of phenytoin serum levels are essential.

5.6.7.7 *Topiramate*

Studies of topiramate in the elderly are very limited, but it has good efficacy and can be safely used. Clearance is reduced in the presence of hepatic or renal impairment. The incidence of central nervous system side effects can be reduced with a slow dose titration. A recommended initial dose is 25mg at night and dosage increments can be made in 25mg steps to an initial maintenance dose of between 50mg/day and 150mg/day in monotherapy.

5.6.7.8 *Valproate*

Valproate is widely used in the elderly, particularly to control generalized tonic-clonic seizures. It is as effective as carbamazepine in this indication. Side effects can vary from those in younger adults and there is an impression that encephalopathic side effects of valproate are common in the elderly. There are pharmacokinetic differences and valproate should be initiated at lower doses than used in young adults. A recommended starting dose is 200mg/day and this should be increased in 200mg increments to an initial maintenance dose of 600mg. There are probably no advantages to the modified release ('chrono') formulation. The drug should not be used if there is evidence of hepatic disease.

5.7 **Epilepsy in children**

The aetiologies, clinical features, and response to treatment of epilepsy of young children differs from adults in a number of ways. Both seizures and antiepileptic drugs affect behaviour, learning, schooling, social, and emotional development. In choosing drug therapy, special attention is needed to cognitive and neurological development. The pharmacokinetics and pharmacodynamics of drug therapy change with age. A detailed description of these topics is outside the scope of this book, but would suffice to say that all children with epilepsy should receive specialist referral.

5.7.1 Social impact of epilepsy

The impact of having epilepsy in children differs in many ways from the impact on adults. Growing up with seizures affects personality development and can interfere with many aspects of everyday life, friendships, schooling, attitudes, parenting, and career choice. The child and family should have access to support and counselling. Children with epilepsy should lead as normal a lifestyle as possible and the common tendency to over-protect (cocoon) children should be discussed and avoided. The social aspects of epilepsy in children are discussed further in Chapter 9.

5.7.2 The type of epilepsy

The range of epilepsy types and syndromes in young children is very different from that in adults. Some of the commoner specific syndromes, and their drug treatment and prognosis, are described in Chapter 2. There are other less common syndromes, which are beyond the scope of this book, and the reader is referred to the further reading section. Where epilepsy occurs with falls (e.g. drop attacks in the Lennox–Gastaut syndrome) special precautions are necessary. These epilepsies inevitably interfere with daily activities and special schooling measures and protection of the head and face by wearing an adequate helmet are often required.

5.7.3 Drug treatment

The pharmacokinetics of drugs change with age. Absorption of antiepileptic drugs is usually faster in infants and young children than in adults. The half-lives of most antiepileptic drugs are prolonged in the first 1–3wks of life and shorten thereafter. The metabolism of antiepileptic drugs is faster during the childhood and slow to adult values during adolescence. Thus, higher doses per unit of weight are required by children, and dose requirements can change over time.

The pharmacodynamic effects of antiepileptic drugs may also differ. The paradoxical effect of barbiturates and benzodiazepines causing excitation in children and sedation in adults is an example. Side effects can be difficult to recognize in infants and in those with learning disability, and the children may not be able to communicate their symptoms. These groups therefore require extra surveillance for side effects. In school aged children, three times daily regimens (requiring dosing at school) should be avoided, as the middle dose is easily overlooked.

Many of the principles for the drug treatment of epilepsy in adults also apply to children—for instance, the use of monotherapy where possible, monitoring of therapy, and restricting dosing to once or twice a day. The choice of drugs will depend on the syndrome, especially in younger children, but in older children it is similar to that in adults.

5.7.4 **The ketogenic diet**

The ketogenic diet is a high-fat and low-carbohydrate diet that was introduced into epilepsy therapy in the 1920s, and which in recent times has been the subject of a resurgence of interest. Its use is confined to the treatment of severe childhood epilepsy which has proved resistant to more conventional therapy. The exact constitution of the diet must be calculated on an individual basis and the effects on epilepsy can be dramatic. A recent study showed, at 1yr, a >50% reduction in seizures in 50% of 150 treated children, and a >90% reduction in 27%. At 3–6yrs, 44% maintained the improvement. The use of the diet allows a reduction of adjunctive drug therapy, which is an added benefit. Side effects are not uncommon. Vomiting, dehydration, and food refusal are common initially but are transitory. Renal stones occur in 5%–8% of patients and hypercholesterolaemia is common. Other minor side effects include constipation, oesophageal reflux, and acidosis. The diet can affect growth (both weight and height) and a recent review of the diet in 237 children showed that the rate of weight gain decreased at 3 months but then remained constant for up to 3yrs.

5.8 **The treatment of epilepsy in women**

There are a number of aspects of therapy that are specific to women with epilepsy.

5.8.1 **Fertility**

Women with epilepsy have approximately 30% fewer pregnancies than their non-epileptic peers. In one study of a general population of 2,052,922 persons in England and Wales, an overall fertility rate was found to be 47.1 (95% CI 42.3–52.2) live births/1,000 women with epilepsy per year compared with a national rate of 62.6. There are potentially a number of varied reasons for this. These include social effects and women with epilepsy have lower rates of marriage and marry later, and suffer social isolation and stigmatization. Pregnancy may be avoided deliberately because of the risk of epilepsy or teratogenicity. Personality or cognitive difficulties may be relevant. Biological effect may also influence fertility rates including genetic factors and the effects of antiepileptic drugs.

5.8.2 **Contraception**

Drugs that induce hepatic enzyme activity (particularly CYP3A family enzymes; barbiturate, phenytoin, primidone, oxcarbazepine, topiramate and carbamazepine) increase the metabolism of the oestrogen and progesterone components of the pill by up to 50% and thereby reduce its efficacy. A higher dose of the pill is therefore needed to achieve contraceptive effect, and the combined contraceptive pill with at least

50mcg oestradiol content or two 30mcg oestradiol pills should be given (note that this is an unlicensed use). Alternatively, 'tricylcing' a 50mcg oestrogen preparation can be employed, which entails taking three monthly packets of the contraceptive without a break, followed by an interval of 4 days rather than the usual 7. Even using higher dose preparations, there is a higher risk of contraceptive failure, and figures of three failures per 1,000 women years are quoted compared to the 0.3/1,000 rate in the general population. There is generally only a small risk with non-CYP3A enzyme-inducing drugs such as vigabatrin, valproate, clobazam, gabapentin, lamotrigine, levetiracetam, and pregabalin. The combined contraceptive pill tends to lower lamotrigine levels by 40%–60%, so starting the pill in patients co-medicated with lamotrigine can result in poorer control and higher drug dosage may be required.

The progesterone only pill (the 'mini-pill') is affected in a similar manner.

The injectable contraceptive, medroxyprogesterone acetate (Depo-Provera®) has no interactions with antiepileptics, as there is virtual 100% clearance on first pass through the level and enzyme induction should have no effect. However, norethisterone enantate long-acting injection and the progestogen implant (Implanon®) are affected by enzyme-inducing drugs, and so should not be used. The intra-uterine contraception (coil) is not affected by drug interactions.

Post-coital contraception (the morning after pill) is also affected by enzyme-inducing antiepileptic drugs, and so the first dose should be doubled and a second single dose given 12hrs later (unlicensed use). An intra-uterine device (IUD) can also be used.

5.8.3 Catamenial epilepsy

Many women have a seizure exacerbation around the time of menstruation. Occasionally seizures only occur at this time, and this pattern is named catamenial epilepsy. Intermittent therapy with acetazolamide or clobazam taken only around the time of menstruation can be tried, although is often unsuccessful.

5.8.4 Risk of seizures during pregnancy

Tonic-clonic seizures occurring during pregnancy do carry a small risk to the developing foetus. Frequent major convulsions have been shown to be associated with a slight increase in the risk of foetal malformation. This risk is probably largely due to mechanical injury, causing, for instance, placental bleeding or premature labour. It seems unlikely that there is significant anoxia or metabolic damage to the foetus during a maternal seizure. The risks of maternal seizures to foetal health therefore are greatest in the last trimester. Nonconvulsive seizures and seizures that do not involve falling or accidental injury probably carry no risk to the foetus. Convulsive status epilepticus is particularly hazardous and carries a significant risk of foetal death.

5.8.5 **Teratogenicity of antiepileptic drugs**

Antiepileptic drugs increase the rate of malformations. The most common major malformations associated with traditional antiepileptic drug therapy (phenytoin, phenobarbital, primidone, benzodiazepine, valproate, carbamazepine) are cleft palate and cleft lip, cardiac malformations, neural tube defects, hypospadias, and skeletal abnormalities. Valproate is associated with a 1%–2% risk, and carbamazepine a 0.5%–1% risk of spina bifida aperta. Both carbamazepine and valproate have also been associated with hypospadias. The overall risk of monotherapy with most drugs, where this is known, lies between 2% and 5% and is slightly higher with valproate. In polytherapy, the risk increases to up to 15% with valproate included in the drug regimen.

In addition to the major malformations, less severe dysmorphic changes ('fetal syndromes') are said to occur, with a characteristic pattern of facial and limb disturbances. Controversy also exists in relation to the question of whether maternal drug usage results in developmental delay and learning disability. A recent study showed that children exposed to valproate monotherapy had significantly lower verbal intelligence quotient (VIQ) scores when compared to children exposed to carbamazepine. Although a connection between subsequent learning disability and valproate therapy is by no means proved, it would be sensible to avoid valproate in pregnancy where possible.

5.8.6 **Drug therapy**

Ideally, a woman's antiepileptic drug regimen should be reviewed before conception to minimize the teratogenic effects of the medication. It is important to establish whether antiepileptic therapy is needed at all. This will be an individual decision, based on the estimated risk of exacerbation of seizures and their danger to both the foetus and the mother. Some women with partial or nonconvulsive seizures will elect to withdraw therapy even if seizures are active or likely to become more frequent. Conversely, some women who are seizure-free will wish to continue therapy because of the social and physical risks of seizure recurrence. In some patients, it is reasonable to withdraw therapy for the first half of pregnancy and then to reinstate the drugs, on the basis most of the major malformations are established within the first trimester of pregnancy and that the risks of seizures are probably greatest in the past trimester.

If the woman elects to continue therapy, the appropriate regimen in most cases is the minimally effective dose of the single antiepileptic that best controls the epilepsy. A few women with severe epilepsy will need combination therapy, but this should be avoided wherever possible. Dose increases may be necessary in later pregnancy as the pharmacokinetics of some drugs can change in pregnancy for various reasons. Levels of lamotrigine may be halved, and levels of phenytoin, phenobarbital, carbamazepine, and valproate can be markedly reduced.

5.8.7 **Effects of epilepsy on pregnancy and delivery**

Approximately three to four live births per 1,000 women of child-bearing age with epilepsy occur each year. The perinatal mortality rate is two times that of the general population. Approximately 1%–2% of all women with epilepsy will have tonic-clonic seizures during delivery and this can clearly complicate labour. Home birth should not generally be contemplated.

5.8.8 **Effect of pregnancy on the rate of seizures**

Pregnancy has a rather random effect on seizure frequency, which improves in approximately one-third of women, remains unchanged in one-third and worsens in one-third. In severe epilepsy, however, seizure frequency is more likely to increase.

5.8.9 **Folic acid supplementation**

All women with epilepsy should take a dose of at least 5mg/day folic acid before and during pregnancy, to lessen the risk of foetal spina bifida.

5.8.10 **New-onset epilepsy during pregnancy**

Seizures starting in pregnancy should be investigated and treated as in non-epileptic patients, although ionizing radiation should be avoided if possible. There is an increased risk of seizures from meningiomas that can grow in size during pregnancy, Arteriovenous malformations that present more commonly in pregnancy, and ischaemic stroke that has a tenfold increased risk in pregnancy. Pregnancy can also predispose to cerebral infections due to bacteria (including *listeria*), fungi (*coccidioides*), protozoa (*toxoplasma*), viruses, and HIV infection.

Most new-onset seizures at the time of delivery are caused by eclampsia. Magnesium has been shown to be more effective in the therapy of eclampsia than phenytoin and/or diazepam. Magnesium sulfate should be administered as an intravenous (IV) infusion of 4g, followed by 5g of 50% solution to each buttock (10g total IM dose) and then 5g every 4hrs as required to alternate buttocks. Magnesium treatment should be continued for 24hrs after delivery or the last convulsion (whichever is last). IM injections should be given with 1ml of 2% lignocaine.

5.8.11 **Breastfeeding**

Most drugs do not enter breast milk in substantial quantities and breastfeeding by a mother taking antiepileptics should be encouraged. However, zonisamide, lamotrigine, phenobarbital, and levetiracetam do enter breast milk. Particular caution is advised in the case of maternal phenobarbital ingestion, as in neonates, the half-life of phenobarbital is long (up to 300hrs) and the free fraction is higher than in adults; neonatal levels can therefore sometimes exceed maternal levels.

References and further reading

Adab N, Tudur SC, Vinten J, Williamson P, and Winterbottom J (2004). Common antiepileptic drugs in pregnancy in women with epilepsy. *Cochrane Database of Systematic Reviews (Online)*, **3**, CD004848.

Arzimanoglou A, Guerrini R, and Aicardi J (2003). *Aicardi's epilepsy in children*, 3rd edn. Lippincott, Williams and Wilkins, Philadelphia.

Benbadis SR and Tatum WO (2003). Overinterpretation of EEGs and misdiagnosis of epilepsy. *Journal of Clinical Neurophysiology*, **20**, 42–4.

Depondt C and Shorvon SD (2006). Genetic association studies in epilepsy pharmacogenomics: lessons learnt and potential applications. *Pharmacogenomics*; **7**, 73145.

Drivers Medical Group, DVLA (2007). *At a glance guide to the current medical standards of fitness to drive*. DVLA, Swansea.

Elger CE, Helmstaedter C, and Kurthen M (2004). Chronic epilepsy and cognition. *Lancet Neurology*, **3**, 663–72.

Engel J and Pedley TA (eds) (2008). *Epilepsy: a comprehensive textbook*, 2nd edn. Raven Press, New York.

French JA, Kanner AM, Bautista J, *et al*. (2004a). Efficacy and tolerability of the new antiepileptic drugs. I: Treatment of new onset epilepsy: report of the Therapeutics and Technology Assessment Subcommittee and Quality Standards Subcommittee of the American Academy of Neurology and the American Epilepsy Society. *Neurology*, **62**, 1252–60.

French JA, Kanner AM, Bautista J, *et al*. (2004b). Efficacy and tolerability of the new antiepileptic drugs. II: Treatment of refractory epilepsy: report of the Therapeutics and Technology Assessment Subcommittee and Quality Standards Subcommittee of the American Academy of Neurology and the American Epilepsy Society. *Neurology*; **62**, 1261–73.

Hart YM, Sander JW, Johnson AL and Shorvon SD (1990). National General Practice Study of Epilepsy: recurrence after a first seizure. *Lancet*, **336**, 1271–4.

Kwan P and Brodie MJ (2004). Phenobarbital for the treatment of epilepsy in the 21st century: a critical review. *Epilepsia*, **45**, 1141–9.

Levy RH, Mattson RH, Meldrum B, and Perucca E (2002). *Antiepileptic drugs*, 5th edn. Lippincott, Williams and Wilkins, Philadelphia.

Luciano AL and Shorvon SD (2007). Results of treatment changes in patients with apparently drug-resistant chronic epilepsy. *Annals of Neurology*, **62**, 375–81.

Marson AG, Al-Kharusi AM, Alwaidh M, *et al*. (2007). The SANAD study of effectiveness of carbamazepine, gabapentin, lamotrigine, oxcarbazepine, or topiramate for treatment of partial epilepsy: an unblended randomized controlled trial. *Lancet*, **369**, 1000–15.

Moran NF, Poole K, Bell G, *et al*. (2004). Epilepsy in the United Kingdom: seizure frequency and severity, antiepileptic drug utilization and impact on life in 1652 people with epilepsy. *Seizure*, **13**, 425–33.

O'Brien MD and Guillebaud J (2006). Contraception for women with epilepsy. *Epilepsia*, **47**, 1419–22.

Patsalos PN and Perucca E (2003a). Clinically important drug interactions in epilepsy: general features and interactions between antiepileptic drugs. *Lancet Neurology*, **2**, 347–56.

Patsalos PN and Perucca E (2003b). Clinically important drug interactions in epilepsy: interactions between antiepileptic drugs and other drugs. *Lancet Neurology*, **2**, 473–81.

Sander JW, Hart YM, Johnson AL, Shorvon SD (1990). National General Practice Study of Epilepsy: newly diagnosed epileptic seizures in a general population. *Lancet*, **336**, 1267–71.

Shorvon S (2006). We live in the age of the clinical guideline. *Epilepsia*, **47**, 1091–3.

Shorvon S (2007). The treatment of chronic epilepsy: a review of recent studies of clinical efficacy and side effects. *Current Opinion in Neurology*, **20**, 159–63.

Shorvon S and Luciano AL (2007). Prognosis of chronic and newly diagnosed epilepsy: revisiting temporal aspects. *Current Opinion in Neurology*, **20**, 208–12.

Shorvon SD (2005). *Handbook of epilepsy treatment: forms, causes and therapy in children and adults.* Blackwell Science, Oxford.

Shorvon SD, Pedley TA (eds) (2009). *The Epilepsies 3*. Vol 33, Blue book of Neurology series. Saunders, Philadelphia.

Shorvon SD, Perucca E, and Engel J (eds) (2009). *The treatment of epilepsy*, 3rd edn. Blackwell Publishing.

Van Paesschen W, Dupont P, Sunaert S, Goffin K, and Van Laere K (2007). The use of SPECT and PET in routine clinical practice in epilepsy. *Current Opinion in Neurology*, **20**, 194–2.

Velis D, Plouin P, Gotman J, da Silva FL, and ILAE DMC Subcommittee on Neurophysiology (2007). Recommendations regarding the requirement and applications for long-term recordings in epilepsy. ILAE Commission Report. *Epilepsia*, **48**, 379–84.

Wallace SJ and Farrell K (eds) (2004). *Epilepsy in children.* Arnold, London.

Zaccara G, Franciotta D, and Perucca E (2007). Idiosyncratic adverse reactions to antiepileptic drugs. *Epilepsia*, **48**, 1223–44.

Chapter 6

Antiepileptic drugs

> **Key points**
> - In the past 20yrs, a large range of antiepileptic drugs have been licensed for use.
> - Only some of these drugs are licensed currently for use in newly diagnosed patients or for use in children.
> - The drugs differ widely in terms of their mechanisms of action, pharmacology, pharmacokinetics, indications, and common and/or important side effects.
> - The physician treating epilepsy should be aware of the main features of all available antiepileptic drugs, and these are summarized in this Chapter.

There are a wide range of antiepileptic drugs available for prescribing. It is important for the practitioner to have a working knowledge of the pharmacology, pharmacokinetics, indications, and common and/or important side effects—and these are summarized in the following sections. Please note, however, that the information is given in outline only, and for further details, please refer to the further reading sections. Other drugs are more rarely given including acetazolamide, felbamate, piracetam, rufinamide, stiripentol and tetracosactide (adrenocorticotropic hormone (ACTH)), and the reader is referred to the 'further reading' section for more details.

Basic pharmacokinetic parameters are shown in Tables 6.1 and 6.2, and the putative mechanisms of actions of the main antiepileptic drugs are shown in Table 6.3.

Table 6.1 Pharmacokinetic parameters of main antiepileptic drugs

Drug	Oral bioavail-ability (%)	Time to peak level (h)	Metabolism	Half-life[a] (h)
Carbamazepine	75–85	4–8	Hepatic	5–26[b]
Clobazam	90	0.5–2	Hepatic	10–45
Clonazepam	85	1–4	Hepatic	17–55
Ethosuximide	~100	1–5	Hepatic	25–70[b]
Gabapentin	~65[d]	2–3	None	5–9
Lacosamide	~100	0.5–4	Hepatic	13
Lamotrigine	~100	1–3	Hepatic	12–60[e]
Levetiracetam	~100	0.5–2	Non-hepatic	6–8
Oxcarbazepine	~100	4–6	Hepatic	8–10[d,b]
Phenobarbital	>95	1–3	Hepatic	75–120[b]
Phenytoin	95	4–12	Hepatic	7–80[b,d]
Pregabalin	90	1–2	None	5–7
Primidone	~100	3	Hepatic	5–18[b] (75–120[1])
Tiagabine	~100	1–2[c]	Hepatic	5–9[b]
Topiramate	~100	2–4	Hepatic	10–30[b]
Valproate	~100	1–10[f]	Hepatic	8–17[b]
Vigabatrin	50	0.5–2	None	4–7
Zonisamide	~100	2–6	Hepatic	50–70[b]

[a] Values for healthy adults.

[b] Half-life varies with co-medication—usually reduced and for some drugs such as lamotrigine, tiagabine, and zonisamide so much so that dose changes are routinely required.

[c] Absorption of tiagabine is markedly slowed by food, and it is recommended that the drug is taken at the end of meals.

[d] Absorption of gabapentin is by a saturable active transport system, and rate will depend on the capacity of the system.

[e] Half-life greatly increased by co-medication with valproate—requiring significant dose reductions.

[f] The time to peak concentration varies according to formulation (0.5–2hrs for normal formulation, 3–8hrs for enteric coated).

Table 6.2 Pharmacokinetic parameters of main antiepileptic drugs

Drug	Protein binding (%)	Active metabolite	Drug interactions
Carbamazepine	75	CBZ-epoxide	a
Clobazam	85–90	N-desmethyl clobazam	b
Clonazepam	86	None	b
Ethosuximide	<10	None	a
Gabapentin	None	None	None
Lacosamide	<15	None	b
Lamotrigine	55	None	a
Levetiracetam	<10	None	b
Oxcarbazepine	38	MHD	a
Phenobarbital	45–60	None	a
Phenytoin	85–95	None	a
Pregabalin	None	None	None
Primidone	25	Phenobarbital	a
Tiagabine	96	None	a
Topiramate	15	None	b
Valproate	70–95	None	a
Vigabatrin	None	None	None
Zonisamide	30–60	None	a

MHD, 10-monohydroxy derivative metabolite.

[a]Many interactions, frequently of clinical relevance and many require dose modification.

[b]Minor interactions, but not usually of much clinical relevance.

Table 6.3 Major putative mechanisms of actions of main antiepileptic drugs

Drug	Major putative mechanisms of action
Carbamazepine	Blocks conductance at the neuronal sodium channel
Clobazam	Enhances GABA action at the GABAergic receptors
Clonazepam	Enhances GABA action at the GABAergic receptors
Ethosuximide	Inhibits neuronal T-type calcium channels
Gabapentin	Binds to the $\alpha2\delta$ subunit of the neuronal voltage-dependent calcium channel
Lacosamide	Enhances selectively slow inactivation at the neuronal sodium channel and modulates the action of the CMRP-2 protein
Lamotrigine	Blocks conductance at the neuronal sodium channel
Levetiracetam	Binds to the synaptic vesicle protein SV2A
Oxcarbazepine	Blocks conductance at the neuronal sodium channel
Phenobarbital	Enhances GABA action at the benzodiazepine site at the GABA$_A$ receptor, inhibits glutamate excitability, weak effect on sodium, potassium, and calcium conductance
Phenytoin	Blocks conductance at the neuronal sodium channel
Pregabalin	Binds to the $\alpha2\delta$ subunit of the neuronal voltage-dependent calcium channel
Primidone	Prodrug of phenobarbital. Mechanism of action same as phenobarbital (see above)
Tiagabine	Enhances GABAergic transmission at the GABA$_A$ receptor by inhibiting GABA re-uptake
Topiramate	Blocks conductance at the neuronal sodium channel, potentiates GABAergic inhibition at the GABA$_A$ receptor, reduces excitatory actions of glutamate at AMPA receptor, inhibits high-voltage calcium channels, inhibits carbonic anhydrase
Valproate	Not fully understood. Action on GABA and glutaminergic activity, calcium (T) conductance, and potassium conductance
Vigabatrin	Enhances GABAergic transmission by inhibiting the catabolic enzyme gamma-aminobutyric acid transaminase (GABA-T), thereby increasing the synaptic concentration of GABA
Zonisamide	Multiple actions including inhibition of sodium and T-type calcium currents, enhances GABAa receptor function, carbonic anhydrase inhibition, glutaminergic transmission inhibition

GABA = gamma-aminobutyric acid.

6.1 **Carbamazepine**

This is an important and a very well-established drug (it has been used in clinical practice since the mid 1960s) and is widely recommended as first-line therapy for partial and secondarily generalized epilepsy. It has for many years been amongst the most widely prescribed drug worldwide. It acts by inhibiting voltage-dependent sodium conductance, with other less significant actions on monoamine, acetylcholine, and N-methyl D-aspartate receptor (NMDA) receptors.

Carbamazepine is very effective and no newer drug has been found in controlled trials to be superior in efficacy in generalized or focal seizures. It is also generally well tolerated although approximately 5% of patients develop a rash on initiation of therapy and everybody should be warned about this. Therapy should be immediately stopped if rash develops, for there is a risk of a Stevens–Johnson reaction. Other side effects are generally worse on initiation of therapy, and this is why the initial dose should be low and later incremented slowly. A slow introduction will avoid side-effects in most patients.

The pharmacokinetics of the drug is not optimal. It is variably and poorly absorbed. Although it has linear kinetics, there is an active metabolite (carbamazepine-10,11-epoxide). Carbamazepine is metabolized in the liver by the CYP3A4 isoform of the P450 enzyme system. Drugs which induce or inhibit CYP3A4 can have marked effects on carbamazepine levels and as carbamazepine is a potent inducer of drug metabolizing enzymes, it also affects the levels of many concomitantly administered drugs.

Box 6.1 Carbamazepine

Usual indication	First-line therapy in partial and generalized tonic-clonic seizures (not absence and myoclonus). Also in some childhood epilepsy syndromes. Adults and children
Preparations	Tablets: 100, 200, 400mg; chewtabs: 100, 200mg; modified-release formulations: 200, 400mg; liquid: 100mg/5mL; suppositories: 125, 250mg
Usual dosage—adults	Starting dose is 100–200mg/day, and increased every 2–3wks by 100/200mg Maintenance dosages are usually in the range of 400–1,600mg/day (Modified-release formulation, give 30% higher dosage.)
Usual dosage—children	<1yr: 100–200mg/day 1–5yrs: 200–400mg/day 5–10yrs: 400–600mg/day 10–15yrs: 600–1,000mg (Modified-release formulation, higher dosage.)
Dosing intervals	2–3 times/day (2–4 times/day at higher doses or in children)
Blood level monitoring	Useful—the usually quoted target range is 17–51µmol/L (4–12mcg/mL)
Common or important side effects	Drowsiness, fatigue, dizziness, ataxia, diplopia, blurring of vision, sedation, headache, insomnia, nausea, loss of appetite, gastrointestinal disturbance, tremor, weight gain, impotence, effects on behaviour and mood, other psychiatric and psychological effects, hepatic disturbance, rash and other skin reactions, bone marrow dyscrasia, changes in blood parameters especially leucopenia, hyponatraemia, water retention, hepatic, renal and endocrine effects, cardiorespiratory effects
Important drug interactions	Carbamazepine is involved in many drug interactions. Amongst the commonest are decrease of carbamazepine levels by concomitant therapy with phenytoin and barbiturates and increase in carbamazepine-10,11-epoxide levels by valproate. Carbamazepine levels can be increased by verapamil, erythromycin, dextropropoxyphene, and many other drugs. Carbamazepine significantly lowers levels of many other antiepileptic drugs and other drugs

6.2 **Clobazam**

Clobazam is an interesting and valuable second-line therapy and has been in clinical use since 1979. It acts as a gamma-aminobutyric acid (GABA)A receptor agonist. It has been licensed since 1984, in Europe (but not in the United States). It is the only commonly used 1,5-benzodiazepine and perhaps as a result of this it has distinctive properties that set it apart from the others. Clobazam is widely felt to be the most useful benzodiazepine by far in chronic treatment. It has a broad-spectrum activity, relatively high response rates in refractory epilepsy, and is generally very well tolerated. It is also used as a one-off therapy for periods of seizure exacerbation (or seizure clusters) and also taken on a single day as prophylaxis on days when the occurrence of a seizure needs to be particularly avoided (e.g. travel, exams, etc.). It is also useful as temporary therapy to provide additional antiepileptic protection during times of drug reduction. The development of tolerance is the main problem with its usage. It is easy to use, without the need for starting at a low dose or dosage incrementation.

Box 6.2 **Clobazam**	
Usual indications	Second-line therapy for partial and generalized tonic-clonic seizures. Also for intermittent therapy, one-off prophylactic therapy and nonconvulsive status epilepticus. Adults and children
Preparations	Tablet: 10mg
Usual dosage—adult	10–20mg/day; higher doses can be used
Usual dosage—children	3–12yrs: 5–10mg/day
Dosing intervals	1–2 times/day
Blood level monitoring	Not usually needed
Common or important side effects	Sedation, dizziness, weakness, blurring of vision, restlessness, ataxia, hypotonia, behavioural disturbance, withdrawal symptoms (especially children)
Important drug interactions	Generally minor, but clobazam clearance is increased by enzyme-inducing agents, and occasionally clobazam may result in an increase in the plasma levels of other antiepileptic drugs

6.3 **Clonazepam**

This is a drug introduced into clinical practice in 1963, now only occasionally used in routine therapy in adults. It has a greater place in severe childhood epilepsies. It has a broad-spectrum action but tolerance and withdrawal seizures limit its value in routine therapy in chronic epilepsy. It is widely used as an effective intravenous (IV) therapy in status epilepticus. Like the other benzodiazepine drugs its main action is as an agonist at the GABA$_A$ receptor.

Box 6.3 Clonazepam	
Usual indications	Second-line therapy in partial and generalized seizures (including absence and myoclonus). Also, in Lennox–Gastaut syndrome, neonatal seizures, infantile spasms, and status epilepticus. Adults and children
Preparations	Tablets: 0.5, 1, 2mg, liquid: 1mg and 2.5mg in 1mL diluent
Usual dosage—adult	Initial: 0.25mg at night Maintenance: 0.5–4mg/day
Usual dosage—children	<1yr: 1mg/day 1–5yrs: 1–2mg/day 5–12yrs: 1–3mg/day
Dosing intervals	1–2 times/day
Blood level monitoring	Not useful
Common or important side effects	Sedation (common and may be severe), cognitive effects, drowsiness, ataxia, personality and behavioural changes, hyperactivity, restlessness, aggressiveness, psychotic reaction, seizure exacerbations, hypersalivation, tone changes, leucopenia, withdrawal symptoms
Important drug interactions	Clonazepam levels can be lowered by co-medication with other enzyme-inducing drugs

6.4 **Ethosuximide**

Ethosuximide was introduced into practice in 1958, and was the first-line therapy of generalized absence seizures for many years. It is now only occasionally used. It acts by blocking conduction in low-voltage activated T-type calcium channels. It is well absorbed, has linear kinetics and is metabolized in the liver (cytochrome CYP3A4). It is only 10% protein bound. Its clearance is reduced by co-medication with valproate. Side effects can be problematic and serious, and include idiosyncratic blood reactions and the induction of behavioural and psychiatric symptoms.

Box 6.4 Ethosuximide	
Usual indications	Generalized absence seizures only. Adults and children
Preparations	Capsules: 250mg; syrup: 250mg/5mL
Usual dosage—adults	Initial: 250mg Maintenance: 750–1500mg/day
Usual dosage—children	Initial: 10–15mg/kg/day Maintenance: 20–40mg/kg/day
Dosing intervals	2–3 times/day
Blood level monitoring	Useful. Target range 40–100mg/L
Common or important side effects	Gastrointestinal symptoms which can be prominent, fatigue, drowsiness, ataxia, diplopia, headache, dizziness, hiccups, sedation, behavioural disturbances including aggression and irritability, hyperexcitability in children, acute psychotic reactions, and other psychiatric side effects especially depression, extrapyramidal symptoms, insomnia, blood dyscrasias of various sorts that can be severe, rash, lupus-like syndrome, and other severe idiosyncratic reactions
Important drug interactions	Ethosuximide levels are reduced by co-medication with carbamazepine, phenytoin, phenobarbital, and other drugs such as rifampicin. Serum valproic acid levels may be decreased by ethosuximide. Ethosuximide levels are increased by some drugs (e.g. isoniazid). Co-medication with ethosuximide does not generally interfere with levels of other antiepileptic drugs

6.5 Gabapentin

Gabapentin was designed to be an analogue of GABA, but in fact its antiepileptic effects are probably due to its binding to the $\alpha2\delta$ subunit of the neuronal voltage-dependent calcium channel. It is used mainly in neurogenic pain, and its epilepsy usage is confined to adjunctive therapy in refractory partial epilepsy. Its place in the therapy of both pain and epilepsy has been to some extent superseded by the newer drug pregabalin, which has the same mechanism of action but is more potent. It has variable absorption, and is poorly absorbed at high doses, but otherwise has excellent pharmacokinetics and is excreted unchanged. It is a well-tolerated drug, but has a reputation of having modest efficacy. It has a role particularly in the treatment of mild epilepsy, in children, or in the elderly where the excellent pharmacokinetics and lack of interactions are a useful feature.

Box 6.5 Gabapentin	
Usual indications	Adjunctive therapy in partial or secondarily generalized epilepsy. Adults and children (over age of 3yrs)
Preparations	Capsules: 100, 300, 400, 600, 800mg 250mg/5ml oral solution
Usual dosage—adult	Initial: 300mg/day Maintenance: 900–3,600mg/day
Usual dosage—children	Initial: 10–15mg/kg/day Maintenance: 40mg/kg/day in children aged 3 and 4yrs, and 25–35mg/kg/day in children 5–12yrs of age
Dosing intervals	2–3 times/day
Blood level monitoring	Not useful
Common or important side effects	Drowsiness, dizziness, weight gain, seizure exacerbation, ataxia, headache, tremor, psychiatric disturbance especially depression and anxiety, cognitive blunting, concentration and memory difficulties, impotence, diplopia, nausea, vomiting, flatulence and other gastrointestinal effects, malaise, asthma, rhinitis, oedema, joint and muscle pains, cough, dyspnoea, itching, pancreatic and hepatic disturbance
Important drug interactions	Nil

6.6 **Lacosamide**

This is the latest antiepileptic drug to be licensed. It has a unique binding site to the CMRP-2 protein, and a novel action on the slow inactivation of the neuronal sodium channel, an action which differs from that of the other conventional antiepileptics acting on the sodium channel such as carbamazepine, phenytoin, or lamotrigine. It shows efficacy in a broad range of experimental epilepsy models. It has excellent pharmacokinetics—complete absorption, linear kinetics, a plasma half-life of approximately 13hrs, dose-level proportionality, low protein bindings. There are no clinically important drug interactions. Clinical trials show the drug to have good efficacy and the long-term retention rate in the open extension of the trials was also very good. It is newly licensed for use as an add-on therapy for partial onset seizures in adults, and its place in routine therapy has not yet been established.

Box 6.6 **Lacosamide**	
Usual indications	Adjunctive therapy for partial-onset seizures with or without secondary generalization. Adults
Preparations	Tablets: 50, 100, 150, 200mg oral syrup: 15mg/mL 10mg/ml solution for infusion
Usual dosage—adult	Initial: 50mg twice daily Maintenance: 200–400mg/day
Dosing intervals	2 times/day
Blood level monitoring	Not useful
Common or important side effects	Reported side-effects are usually mild and transient. The most common include: dizziness, headache, nausea, diplopia and fatigue. Other common side effects include blurring of vision, asthenia, gait disturbance, depression, balance disorder, memory disturbance, tremor, vertigo, vomiting, constipation, pruritis.
Important drug interactions	It has no effect on the plasma levels of other drugs. Co-medication with other enzyme-inducing drugs may reduce the lacosamide level slightly

6.7 Lamotrigine

This drug was first licensed for use in 1991. It has since established a place as a useful first- and second-line therapy in a broad spectrum of epilepsies. It acts by blocking sodium channel conduction, like phenytoin and carbamazepine. It has complex pharmacokinetics, is metabolized in the liver, and has drug interactions that complicate its use. The most important interaction is with valproate, co-medication with which can result in a very marked elevation of lamotrigine levels. Hypersensitivity can occur, with severe effects on blood and skin. A troublesome side effect is an allergic rash which can be occasionally severe or progress to a Stevens–Johnson syndrome. The frequency of skin rash is higher in children than in adults (early reports suggested that 1 in 50 children developed a potentially life-threatening rash, but the incidence has fallen since the recognition that slow incrementation particularly in patients co-medicated with valproate greatly reduces the risk. The impact of side effects is generally low, although some side effects such as insomnia are common and can limit its use. In the later stages of pregnancy, the levels of lamotrigine can fall greatly. Its main disadvantages relate to the need to individualize dose according to co-medication and the need for a slow introduction of therapy. Its main advantages are its broad spectrum and relatively good tolerability.

Table 6.4 Dosing of lamotrigine in children

Adjunctive therapy with valproate:	
Children 2–12 yrs	• initially 150mcg/kg/daily • maintenance 1-5mg/kg/day
Children 12–18 yrs	• initially 25mg alt die • maintenance 100-200mg/day
Adjunctive therapy with enzyme inducing drugs but without valproate:	
Children 2–12 yrs	• initially 600 mcg/day • maintenance 5-15mg/kg/day
Children 12–18 yrs	• initially 50mg/day • maintenance 200-400mg/day (up to a max. of 700mg/day)
Monotherapy:	
Children 12–18 yrs	• initially 25mg/day • maintenance 100-400mg/day (up to a maximum of 500mg/day)

Box 6.7 Lamotrigine

Usual indications	First-line or adjunctive therapy in partial and generalized epilepsy. Also in Lennox–Gastaut syndrome and other generalized epilepsy syndromes. Adults and children
Preparations	Tablets: 25, 50, 100, 150mg, 200mg; dispersible chewable tablets 2, 5, 25, 100mg
Usual dosage—adult	Initial: 12.5–25mg/day Maintenance depends on co-medication: • Combination therapy without valproate and without enzyme-inducing agents: 200–400mg/day—initial monotherapy: 100–200mg/day • Combination therapy with valproate without enzyme-inducing agents: 100–200mg/day • Combination therapy with enzyme-inducing agents without valproate: 300–500mg/day
Usual dosage—children	Initial dosage and maintenance depends on co-medication and on age. Highest doses are needed in children taking enzyme-inducing drugs and lowest doses in those co-medicated with valproate alone. Intermediate doses are recommended in monotherapy or in those co-medicated with oxcarbazepine alone, or with a mixture of valproate and enzyme-inducing drugs. See Table 6.4 and package insert or formulary for details.
Dosing intervals	2 times/day
Blood level monitoring	Of limited usefulness. Usual target range 2.5–15mg/L
Common or important side effects	Rash and hypersensitivity reaction involving fever, hepatic dysfunction, blood dyscrasia DIC and multi-organ failure (this hypersensitivity reaction is sometimes severe and can be life-threatening), headache, ataxia, asthenia, fatigue, diplopia, nausea, vomiting, dizziness, somnolence, insomnia, depression, psychosis, tremor, movement disorder, other neurological and psychiatric effects, arthralgia, lupus-like syndrome and photosensitivity
Important drug interactions	Serum lamotrigine levels are reduced by many drugs, including enzyme-inducing antiepileptic drugs (e.g. carbamazepine, phenytoin, phenobarbital), rifampicin, combined steroid contraceptives. Serum lamotrigine levels are markedly increased by valproic acid. Lamotrigine may reduce the serum levels of levonorgestrel

6.8 **Levetiracetam**

The drug was licensed in 1999/2000 in the United States/Europe and is a powerful antiepileptic compound, which has rapidly gained an important place in clinical practice both in monotherapy and poly-therapy. It has excellent pharmacokinetics and is metabolized largely by hydrolysis. Only 24% of the drug is metabolized in the liver. Co-medication with levetiracetam does not affect levels of other drugs, although enzyme-inducing drugs can lower levetiracetam levels. Dosage needs to be reduced in renal disease. It is easy to use in clinical practice and has a broad-spectrum activity in epilepsy, controlling generalized and partial seizures. It is generally very well tolerated without the usual sedative effects of other antiepileptic drugs. Its main drawback is its tendency in susceptible individuals to cause marked irritability and occasionally aggressive or psychotic behaviour. It can paradoxically increase seizure frequency in occa-sional patients especially at high doses. It acts by binding to the synaptic vesicle (SV2A) protein and this is a unique mode of action not shared by other widely used antiepileptics.

Its current licensing is as adjunctive therapy for partial seizures in adults and children from 4yrs of age; adjunctive therapy for myoclonic seizures in adults and adolescents with juvenile myoclonic epilepsy from 12yrs of age; as adjunctive therapy for primary generalized tonic-clonic seizures in adults and adolescents with idiopathic gener-alized epilepsy (IGE) from 12yrs of age in Europe and from 6yrs of age in the United States; initial monotherapy for partial seizures in adults, in Europe but not in the United States.

Box 6.8 Levetiracetam

Usual indications	First-line and adjunctive therapy of partial-onset seizures and of generalized tonic-clonic seizures and myoclonic seizures in idiopathic generalized epilepsy (IGE). May also be useful for other generalized seizure types
Preparations	Tablets: 250, 500, 750, 1,000mg Oral solution: 100mg/mL IV: 500mg/5mL
Usual dosage—adult	Initial: 125–250mg/day, with increments of 125–250mg every 2 weeks Maintenance: 750–3,000mg/day
Usual dosage—children	Initial: 10–20mg/kg/day with increments of 10–20mg/kg/day every 2 weeks. Maintenance: 20–60mg/kg/day
Dosing intervals	2 times/day
Serum level monitoring	Occasionally useful. Target range 12–46mg/L
Common or important side effects	Behavioural change, irritability, aggression, mood change, depression, anxiety, psychosis, dizziness, headache, unsteadiness, tremor and hyperkinesis, memory and attention disturbance, somnolence, asthenia, visual disturbance, gastrointestinal disturbance, infection, itching, rash, alopecia, blood dyscrasia, myalgia, pancreatic and hepatic disturbance, cough
Important drug interactions	Interactions are seldom a problem, but levetiracetam levels can fall by up to 20%–30% on co-medication with carbamazepine

6.9 **Oxcarbazepine**

Oxcarbazepine is the 10-keto analogue of carbamazepine. It was introduced into clinical practice in Denmark in 1990, but licensed in other EU countries in 1999 and in the United States in 2000. Oxcarbazepine is metabolized first by reduction, avoiding the oxidative step that carbamazepine undergoes and thus the production of the oxidative metabolite of carbamazepine (CBZ-epoxide) that is responsible for some carbamazepine side effects. The pharmacological action of oxcarbazepine is exerted almost exclusively through its active 10-monohydroxy derivative metabolite (MHD).

Its antiepileptic effects are very similar to those of carbamazepine, and its mode of action is identical. It has fewer and less marked drug interactions. Side effects are also similar although it is generally somewhat better tolerated than carbamazepine. It has, however, a more marked propensity to cause hyponatraemia which can be severe. Although the risk of serious rash is lower with carbamazepine, a mild skin rash is relatively common (approximately 5%–10% of all patients). Approximately 25%–30% of those experiencing a serious rash or hypersensitivity on carbamazepine will also experience hypersensitivity to oxcarbazepine.

Box 6.9 Oxcarbazepine

Usual indications	First- or second-line treatment in partial and secondarily generalized seizures Adults and children
Preparations	Tablets: 150, 300, 600mg Oral suspension 300mg/ml
Usual dosage—adult	Initial: 300mg/day Maintenance: 900–2,400mg/day
Usual dosage—children	Initial: 4–5mg/kg/day, increased by increments of 5mg/kg/day weekly Maintenance: 20–45mg/kg/day
Dosing intervals	2 times/day
Serum level monitoring	Useful in some cases. Target range 3–35mg/L
Common or important side effects	The side effect profile is very similar to carbamazepine (see preceding text). The commonest side effects are dizziness, unsteadiness, diplopia, ataxia, somnolence, headache, fatigue, nausea, gastrointestinal disturbances. Rash and hypersensitivity reactions which can be severe. Hyponatraemia is more common and more marked than on carbamazepine. Other side effects include anorexia, alopecia, pancreatic disturbance, lupus-like syndrome, cardiorespiratory disturbance, and other cognitive and neurological symptoms
Important drug interactions	Fewer interactions than with carbamazepine. Enzyme-inducing antiepileptic drugs reduce the serum levels of the active metabolite MHD. Oxcarbazepine co-medication increases serum levels of phenytoin and phenobarbital, and reduces serum levels of oral contraceptives

6.10 Phenobarbital

Phenobarbital is a remarkable compound, introduced into practice in 1912, and still, in volume terms, the most commonly prescribed antiepileptic drug in the world. It is by far the cheapest of the antiepileptic drugs commonly available. It is highly effective with an efficacy, which generally speaking has not been much exceeded by any subsequent drug. It is extensively metabolized in the liver and is involved in a number of drug interactions although these are usually minor. It has a very long half-life and a tendency to accumulate. Its main disadvantages relate to its cerebral side effects and its tendency to cause sedation, but this is seldom a problem at low doses. In children, there is a strong tendency to cause hyperexcitability and behavioural change, which limits its use. Its main mechanism of action in enhancement of GABA$_A$ receptor activity, but it also depresses glutamate excitability and affects sodium, potassium, and calcium conductance. It remains a drug of choice in neonatal seizures and in the treatment of status epilepticus.

Box 6.10 Phenobarbital	
Usual indications	First- or second-line therapy for partial or generalized seizures (including absence and myoclonus). Lennox–Gastaut syndrome. Other childhood epilepsy syndromes, febrile convulsions, neonatal seizures and status epilepticus
Preparations	Tablets: 15, 30, 50, 60, 100mg; Liquid: 15mg/5mL; injection: 200mg/mL
Usual dosage—adults	Initial: 30mg/day. Increments of 30mg every 2 weeks Maintenance: 30–180mg/day
Usual dosage—children	Neonates: 3–4mg/kg//day Children 1 month–12 years: initially 1 to 1.5mg/kg twice daily, increased by 2mg/kg daily as required; usual maintenance dose 2.5–4mg/kg once or twice a day. Children 12–18yrs: 30–180mg/day
Dosing intervals	1–2 times/day
Serum level monitoring	Useful in some patients. Target range 10–40mg/L
Common or important side effects	Rash and other idiosyncratic reactions. Sedation, lethargy, somnolence, headache, dizziness, diplopia, ataxia, rash, hyponatraemia, weight gain, alopecia, nausea, gastrointestinal disturbance. Aggressiveness, cognitive dysfunction, impotence, reduced libido, paradoxical hyperkinesis and behavioural change in children. Psychiatric effects including depression. Cognitive effects including memory and attentional disturbances, Folate and vitamins D and K deficiency, Dupuytren's contracture, frozen shoulder, other connective tissue and cosmetic effects, osteopenia and osteomalacia
Important drug interactions	Phenobarbital is a potent hepatic enzyme inducer and stimulates the metabolism of many other drugs including antiepileptics. Serum phenobarbital levels are also reduced because of induction by many other drugs, and increased due to inhibition by the co-administration of drugs such as valproate

6.11 **Phenytoin**

Phenytoin was introduced into clinical practice in 1938. Although no longer considered first-line therapy in Europe, it remains one of the most widely used antiepileptic drugs in the world because of its low cost and strong antiepileptic effect.

It has difficult pharmacokinetic properties, with non-linear kinetics, extensive hepatic metabolism, and many drug interactions. Because of this, its use requires regular serum level monitoring especially when changing therapy. Once a satisfactory phenytoin dosage regimen has been achieved in a particular patient, it will rarely be necessary to alter that regimen over many years. The list of side effects is long but most patients on chronic therapy do not experience marked side effects, and there is no strong evidence of any general difference in tolerability between phenytoin and other old (or new) drugs. It is now usually reserved as a drug of second choice in partial and secondarily generalized seizures, and also in primary generalized tonic-clonic seizures. Its major mechanism of action, as with carbamazepine, is mediated by inhibition of voltage-dependent sodium channels. It is a drug of choice in the treatment of status epilepticus.

Box 6.11 Phenytoin

Usual indications	First- or second-line therapy in partial and primary and secondarily generalized seizures (excluding myoclonus and absence)
Preparations	Capsules: 25, 30, 50, 100, 200mg; chewtabs: 50mg; liquid suspension: 30mg/5mL, 125mg/50mL; injection: 250mg/5mL
Usual dosage—adult	Initial: 200mg at night Maintenance: 200–500mg/day (higher doses can be used; guided by serum level monitoring)
Usual dosage—children	Child 1 month–12 yrs: initially 1.5–2.5mg/kg twice daily, then adjusted according to response and plasma-phenytoin concentration to 2.5–5mg/kg twice daily (usual max. 7.5mg/kg twice daily or 300mg daily) Child 12–18yrs: initially 75–150mg twice daily then adjusted according to response and plasma-phenytoin concentration to 150–200mg twice daily (usual max. 300mg twice daily)
Dosing intervals	1–2 times/day
Serum level monitoring	Mandatory. Target range is 40–80µmol/L (10–20mg/L)
Common or important adverse events	Hypersensitivity comprising rash, fever, hepatic and renal disturbance, a lupus-like syndrome, lymphadenopathy, and a variety of blood dyscrasias (this hypersensitivity reaction can be severe). Ataxia, dizziness, lethargy, sedation, psychiatric disturbance including depression and anxiety and psychosis, headache, dyskinesia, acute encephalopathy (phenytoin intoxication), insomnia, tremor, psychological changes including memory and attentional defects, connective tissue alterations, gingival hyperplasia, coarsened facies, hirsutism, osteopenia and osteomalacia, vitamins D and K and folate deficiency, megaloblastic anaemia, hypocalcaemia, hormonal dysfunction, loss of libido, pseudolymphoma, hepatitis, coagulation defects, bone marrow hypoplasia, gastrointestinal disturbance including nausea and vomiting and anorexia, weight change, cardiorespiratory changes, polyarteritis nodosa, lupus-like syndrome, interstitial nephritis, pneumonitis
Important drug interactions	Phenytoin is a strong enzyme inducer and reduces the serum levels of many other drugs. Similarly, numerous drugs interfere with phenytoin absorption, plasma protein binding, and metabolism

111

6.12 **Pregabalin**

Pregabalin was licensed as an antiepileptic drug in 2004 for adjunctive use in partial seizures in adults, both in the Unites States and in Europe. In addition to its epilepsy indications, it is licensed as an analgesic for neuropathic pain. It is structurally similar to gabapentin and acts in the same way, by modulating neurotransmitter release by binding to the α2-δ subunit of voltage-gated calcium channels. It has excellent pharmacokinetics and is excreted largely unchanged and has no drug interactions. These are significant advantages in many clinical situations. It also has a mild anxiolytic effect. Its main side effects are weight gain and central nervous system (CNS) effects such as sedation and these tend to be dose-related and may be dose-limiting. It is a powerful antiepileptic and a useful addition to second-line therapy.

Box 6.12 **Pregabalin**	
Usual indications	Second-line therapy for partial seizures with or without secondary generalization. Adults only
Preparations	Capsules: 25, 50, 75, 100, 150, 200, 225, 300mg
Usual dosage—adult	Initial: 50mg/day, with increments of 50mg every 2 weeks Maintenance: 150–600mg/day
Dosing intervals	2 times/day
Serum level monitoring	Not routinely needed
Common or important side effects	Dizziness, somnolence, ataxia, asthenia, increased appetite and weight gain, visual disturbances, tremor, memory and attentional deficit, confusion and other cognitive effects, psychiatric disturbance, change in sexual function, blurred vision, peripheral oedema, dry mouth, gastrointestinal disturbances, flatulence, cardiorespiratory disturbance, myalgia, joint pains, hepatic and pancreatic disturbance. Rare cases of hypersensitivity have been reported including severe skin reactions and blood dyscrasia
Important drug interactions	Nil

6.13 **Primidone**

Primidone is a 'prodrug' of phenobarbital, introduced into clinical practice in 1952, and its action is probably entirely due to the derived phenobarbital. It has no clinical advantage (and significant disadvantages) compared to phenobarbital, although it is not, like phenobarbital, a drug of abuse and therefore not subject to special controls. The side effects are the same as those of phenobarbital, with the additional problem of a propensity to cause intense dizziness, nausea, and sedation at the onset of therapy (sometimes after only one tablet) if the dose started is too high. These effects are probably due to the initially high concentration of the parent drug and disappear after a week or so. Because of this reaction it is always advisable to start primidone at a very low dose.

Box 6.13 Primidone	
Usual indications	As for phenobarbital
Preparations	Tablet, 250mg; suspension: 50mg/mL
Usual dosage—adult	Initial: 62.5–125mg/day. Increased by 125–250mg increments every 2 weeks Maintenance: 500–1,500mg/day
Usual dosage—children	Initial: 25mg increased gradually. Maintenance: 10–25mg/kg/day
Dosing intervals	2 times/day
Serum level monitoring	It is useful to measure the derived phenobarbital levels
Common or important adverse events	As for phenobarbital. Also, dizziness, nausea, and sedation at the initiation of therapy if dose is too high
Important drug interactions	As for phenobarbital

6.14 **Tiagabine**

Tiagabine was introduced into clinical practice in 1998 as adjunctive therapy in refractory patients with partial or secondarily generalized seizures, in adults and in children over the age of 12yrs. It is a GABA re-uptake blocker, and acts by enhancing GABAergic transmission. This is a mechanism of action similar to that of vigabatrin but tiagabine does not carry the risk of psychosis and depression or the visual field defects, which are major side effects of vigabatrin. It is metabolized by the hepatic cytochrome CYP3A4 enzymes, is 96% protein bound, and has a half-life of 5–9hrs but which is reduced to 2–4hrs in co-medication with enzyme-inducing drugs. Its use, however, is complicated by the need to titrate slowly, the potential for drug interactions which result in the need for dose changes, and the frequent need for three or even four times a day dosing. It should always be taken with food, and preferably at the end of meals, to avoid rapid increase in plasma concentrations—and giving with food will greatly improve tolerability. Individual dosing four times daily may also be helpful, at least with higher doses. Minor dose-related side effects are common but the frequency of idiosyncratic drug-related reactions, including cutaneous reactions, is very low. It has a strong tendency to exacerbate seizures in the generalized epilepsies, and to precipitate nonconvulsive status epilepticus. It has generally only a small role in contemporary therapy.

Box 6.14 **Tiagabine**	
Usual indications	Adjunctive therapy in partial and secondarily generalized seizures. Patients ≥12yrs of age only
Preparations	Tablets 2.5, 5, 10, 15mg in Europe: 2, 4, 12, 16mg, in the United States and Canada
Usual dosage—adult	Initial: 4–5mg/day. Slow increase by increments of 4–5mg/week Maintenance: 15–30mg/day (30–45mg/day in co-medication with enzyme-inducing drugs)
Dosing intervals	3 times a day
Serum level monitoring	Not needed
Common or important side effects	Dizziness, tiredness, nervousness, tremor, diarrhoea, nausea, headache, ataxia, confusion, psychosis, depression, word-finding difficulties and other cognitive effects, emotional lability, flu-like symptoms, gastrointestinal disturbances, and exacerbation especially of myoclonic and absence seizures and the precipitation of nonconvulsive status epilepticus
Important drug interactions	Most enzyme-inducing antiepileptic drugs increase tiagabine clearance by stimulating its metabolism and dose changes often needed

6.15 **Topiramate**

Topiramate was licensed in the United Kingdom in 1994 and subsequently in the United States and Europe and many countries worldwide. It is a sulfamate-substituted monosaccharide with various mechanisms of action, which include inhibition of voltage-gated sodium channels, potentiation of GABA-mediated inhibition at the GABA$_A$ receptor, reduction of α-amino-3-hydroxyl-5-methyl-4-isoxazole-propionate (AMPA) receptor activity, inhibition of high-voltage calcium channels, and carbonic anhydrase activity. Its pharmacokinetic properties are generally favourable, although it is metabolized in the liver and can be involved in drug interactions, albeit usually of a minor nature. It has gained a reputation as a powerful antiepileptic drug effective in some patients in whom all other medications have failed. It is effective in a broad spectrum of epilepsies, but has a particular place in the treatment of resistant focal seizures, and symptomatic generalized epilepsies. The early clinical trials were carried out at higher doses than are now currently recommended, and although these studies showed marked efficacy, the rate of neurological and cognitive side effects was also high. However, subsequent experience shows that lower doses are also effective and confer better tolerability, and in routine practice now, the rate of side effects is lower than initially feared. The risk of side effects can also be greatly reduced by starting the drug at a very low dose and titrating upwards slowly.

Box 6.15 Topiramate

Usual indications	Adjunctive therapy or monotherapy in partial and secondarily generalized seizures. Also useful for Lennox–Gastaut syndrome and primary generalized tonic-clonic seizures Adults and children over 2yrs of age
Preparations	Tablets: 25, 50, 100, 200mg; sprinkle capsules: 15, 25, 50mg
Usual dosage—adult	Initial: 25–50mg/day increasing in 25mg increments every 2 weeks Maintenance: 75–400mg/day
Usual dosage—children	Initial: 0.5–1mg/kg/day Maintenance: monotherapy 2–6mg/kg/day Adjunctive therapy 2–9mg/kg/day. High doses can be used, guided by clinical outcome
Dosing intervals	2 times/day
Serum level monitoring	Helpful in occasional cases. Target level 5–20mg/L
Common or important side effects	Dizziness, ataxia, headache, parasthesia, tremor, somnolence, visual blurring, cognitive dysfunction especially difficulties with memory, attention, language and word finding, confusion, agitation, amnesia, depression, anxiety, psychosis, emotional lability, diplopia, loss of appetite and weight loss (which can be marked), nausea, abdominal pain, taste disturbance, dyspepsia, acidosis, and alopecia. Hypersensitivity reaction involving blood, skin, and liver has been very rarely reported
Important drug interactions	Interactions are generally slight. However, topiramate levels can be lowered by co-medication with carbamazepine, phenobarbital, and phenytoin. Topiramate co-medication can increase phenytoin levels

6.16 Valproate

Valproate was licensed in Europe in the early 1960s and then in the United States in 1978. It is manufactured as sodium, magnesium or calcium salts, valproic acid and also as semisodium valproate (Depakote®) which is also known as divalproex sodium (USAN). Its mechanisms of action have not been fully established, but it has effects on GABA and glutaminergic activity, calcium (T) conductance and potassium conductance. Sodium valproate is the usual form in the United Kingdom and Depakote® in Europe. Valpromide (dipropy-lacetamide), a prodrug of valproate, is also marketed, as is a delayed-release formulation of sodium valproate. The term valproate is usually adopted to refer to all these forms. Although properties vary to some extent, none of these formulations have been shown to confer any real superiority over the others. Valproate is still one of the most commonly used antiepileptics throughout the world. It is a drug of first choice in all seizure types (absence, myoclonus, tonic-clonic) in *Idiopathic Generalized Epilepsy* and is strikingly more effective than lamotrigine, topiramate, and barbiturate drugs in this syndrome. Whether levetiracetam can compete with its effectiveness is not yet clear. It is also a drug of first choice in the *Lennox–Gastaut syndrome* where it controls atypical absence and atonic seizures better than most other first-line drugs. It is also a drug of first choice in the syndromes of myoclonic epilepsy and the *Progressive Myoclonic Epilepsies*, and for epilepsies with photosensitivity and/or generalized spike-wave electrographically. In partial and secondarily generalized epilepsy, carbamazepine is usually tried before valproate, although there is no real evidence that valproate is less effective in new or mild cases.

Side effects remain a problem. Weight gain is common and often problematic. Other side effects, such as the neurotoxic effects and effects on hair growth are also common, but often only slight and usually are not a reason for drug withdrawal. In female patients, the possibility that valproate increases the frequency of polycystic ovaries, cause menstrual irregularities, and reduce fertility are enough for many to avoid its use although scientific evidence on these points is generally slight. Valproate teratogenicity is a major concern and is a further reason for avoiding valproate in female patients where pregnancy is an issue. Its use in young children, especially those under 2yrs of age, carries a small but definite risk of hepatic failure and where other drugs are available these tend now to be used. It is contraindicated in the presence of hepatic or pancreatic disease. Valproate pharmacokinetics are complex and there are many and varied interactions. It slightly inhibits the metabolism of other antiepileptic drugs, usually without consequence, but does cause major rises in lamotrigine levels when given as co-medication. Imipenem antibiotics profoundly lower valproate levels and should not be used in co-medication.

Valproate concentrations are lowered by co-medication with commonly used cytotoxic drugs and elevated by co-medication with commonly used antidepressant and psychotropic drugs.

Box 6.16 Valproate	
Usual indication	First- or second- line therapy in all forms of epilepsy at all age groups
Preparations	Enteric-coated tablets: 200, 500mg; crushable tablets: 100mg; capsules: 150, 300, 500mg; solution or syrup: 200mg/5mL, 250mg/5mL; sustained-release tablets: 200, 300, 500mg; sustained-release microspheres, sachets: 100, 250, 500, 750, 1,000mg; divalproex tablets: 125, 300, 500mg (as valproic acid equivalents); divalproex tablets delayed release: 125, 250, 500mg (as valproic acid equivalents); divalproex sprinkles, 125mg (as valproic acid equivalents); divalproex tablets extended release: 250, 500mg (as valproic acid equivalents); solution for IV injection: 100mg/mL
Usual dosage—adult	Initial: 200–500mg/day increasing by 200–500mg increments every 2 weeks Usual maintenance doses: 600–2,000mg/day
Usual dosage—children	Neonates: initially 20mg/kg once daily; usual maintenance dose 20mg/kg Child 1 month–12yrs: initially 10–15mg/kg; usual maintenance dose 25–30mg/kg twice daily (up to 60mg/kg in infantile spasms; monitor clinical chemistry and haematological parameters if dose exceeds 20mg/kg twice daily
Dosing intervals	2–3 times/day
Serum level monitoring	Levels show marked diurnal variation, but can be useful in occasional cases. Target range is 50–100mg/L
Common or important side effects	Nausea, vomiting, hyperammonaemia and other metabolic effects, endocrine effects, weight gain, severe hepatic toxicity, gastrointestinal disturbance, pancreatitis, drowsiness, cognitive disturbance, aggressiveness, tremor, ataxia, weakness, encephalopathy, extrapyramidal symptoms, oedema, thrombocytopenia, neutropenia, platelet and coagulation dysfunction, aplastic anaemia, hair thinning and hair loss, polycystic ovarian syndrome, Fanconi syndrome, hyponatraemia
Important drug interactions	Enzyme-inducing drugs can reduce serum levels, and sometimes markedly so (especially the meropenem antibiotics). Other drugs, such as isoniazid, can increase valproate levels. Valproate inhibits the metabolism of a number of drugs, most notably phenobarbital, lamotrigine, and rufinamide. Valproate displaces phenytoin from plasma protein binding sites and can also inhibit phenytoin metabolism.

6.17 Vigabatrin

Vigabatrin is a GABA agonist, which was introduced in 1989 for the treatment of parietal seizures. It was then noted in 1997 to cause visual field constriction, a side effect which is now known to occur in over 40% of treated patients. Because of this, its use has become severely restricted to a very small number of patients with partial epilepsy whose seizures are controlled with no other available antiepileptic drug. It also has other significant side effects including depression and psychosis. It has a strong effect in infantile spasms, and is often effective in cases resistant to ACTH and because of this has also become a drug of first choice in this small indication. It is particularly effective in cases in which the infantile spasms are due to tuberous sclerosis.

Box 6.17 Vigabatrin	
Usual indications	Adjunctive therapy in partial epilepsy, but only if uncontrolled and supervised by specialist. First-line therapy of infantile spasms
Preparations	Tablets: 500mg; powder 500mg/sachet
Usual dosage—adult	Initial: 500mg increasing by 500mg increments to 2–3g/day
Usual dosage—children	Maintenance: 10–15kg: 0.5–1g/day; 15–30kg:1–1.5g/day; 30–50kg: 1.5–3g/day
Dosing intervals	2 times/day
Serum level monitoring	Not useful
Common or important side effects	Nausea, other gastrointestinal disturbances, abdominal pain, drowsiness, dizziness, encephalopathy, psychosis, depression, stupor, confusion, irreversible visual field restriction, blurred vision, ataxia, weight gain, headache, tremor, parasthesia, exacerbation of myoclonic and other generalized seizure types, nonconvulsive status epilepticus
Important drug interactions	None

6.18 **Zonisamide**

Zonisamide is a chemically distinctive sulfonamide drug, with striking effectiveness in a wide spectrum of partial and generalized seizures. It has been licensed in Japan for some years, although has become available in Europe only since 2002. The drug may have a particular role in the *Progressive Myoclonic Epilepsies*. It has multiple potential mechanisms of action. Zonisamide Inhibits voltage-gated sodium channel and T-type calcium channel currents, acts to enhance the benzodiazepine GABA$_A$ receptor, is a carbonic anhydrase, and also has actions on excitatory glutaminergic transmission. It is prone to cause various side effects and tolerability can be improved by slow introduction. The risk of renal stones has been a concern particularly in Europe and the United States, but less so in Japan and patients should be advised to remain well hydrated when taking this drug. It has approximately 50% protein binding and a very long half-life (50–70hrs) but this is significantly reduced (25–40hrs) by co-medication with enzyme-inducing antiepileptic drugs and changes in dose in co-medication are needed.

Box 6.18 Zonisamide	
Usual indications	Adjunctive therapy in partial and generalized epilepsy (all types). Lennox–Gastaut syndrome. West syndrome. Progressive myoclonic epilepsy. Licensed in Japan and Asia in children and adults. Licensed in the USA and Europe only for refractory partial epilepsy in patients ≥16yrs of age
Preparations	Capsules: 25, 50, 100mg
Usual dosage—adult	Initial dose: 50mg/day initially, increased by 50mg increments each 2 weeks Maintenance: 200–500mg/day
Usual dosage— children	Initial: 2–4mg/kg/day Maintenance: 4–8mg/kg/day
Dosing intervals	1–2 times/day
Serum level monitoring	Useful in many cases. Target range 10–40mg/L
Common or important adverse events	Somnolence, ataxia, dizziness, insomnia, headache, attention and concentration difficulties, memory impairment, irritability, confusion, depression, impaired concentration, mental slowing, speech disturbance, fatigue, nausea, vomiting, weight loss, anorexia, itching, abdominal pain, hyperthermia, nephrolithiasis, acidosis, pyrexia, renal impairment, oligohidrosis, heat intolerance, and risk of heat stroke. Rash and other manifestations of hypersensitivity are rare but can be serious
Important drug interactions	Serum zonisamide levels are markedly lowered by carbamazepine, phenytoin, and barbiturates. Zonisamide co-medication does not usually significantly influence levels of other drugs

References and further reading

Engel J and Pedley TA (eds) (2008). *Epilepsy: a comprehensive textbook*, 2nd edn. Raven Press, New York.

Chadwick D, Marson T (2007). Choosing a first drug treatment for epilepsy after SANAD: randomized controlled trials, systematic reviews, guidelines and treating patients. *Epilepsia*, **48**, 1259–63.

French JA, Kanner AM, Bautista J, Abou-Khalil B, Browne T, Harden CL, *et al* (2004). Efficacy and tolerability of the new anti-epileptic drugs, I: Treatment of new-onset epilepsy: report of the TTA and QSS Subcommittees of the American Academy of Neurology and the American Epilepsy Society. *Epilepsia*, **45**, 401–9.

French JA, Kanner AM, Bautista J, Abou-Khalil B, Browne T, Harden CL, *et al* (2004). Efficacy and tolerability of the new anti-epileptic drugs, II: Treatment of refractory epilepsy: report of the TTA and QSS Sub-committees of the American Academy of Neurology and the American Epilepsy Society. *Epilepsia*, **45**, 410–23.

Glauser T, Ben-Menachem E, Bourgeois B, Cnaan A, Chadwick D, Guerreiro C, *et al* (2006). ILAE treatment guidelines: evidence-based analysis of anti-epileptic drug efficacy and effectiveness as initial monotherapy for epileptic seizures and syndromes. *Epilepsia*, **47**, 1094–120.

Levy RH, Mattson RH, Meldrum B, and Perucca E (2002). *Anti-epileptic drugs*, 5th edn. Lippincott, Williams and Wilkins, Philadelphia.

Panayiotopoulos CP (2007) Evidence-based epileptology, randomized controlled trials,and SANAD: a critical clinical view. *Epilepsia*, **48**, 1268–74.

Patsalos PN, Berry DJ, Bourgeois BF, Cloyd JC, Glauser TA, Johannessen SI, *et al* (2008) Anti-epileptic drugs—best practice guidelines for therapeutic drug monitoring: a position paper by the subcommission on therapeutic drug monitoring, ILAE Commission on Therapeutic Strategies. *Epilepsia*, **49**, 1239–76.

Shorvon SD (2006) We live in the age of the clinical guideline. *Epilepsia*, **47**, 1091–3.

Shorvon SD, Perucca E, and Engel J (eds) (2009). *The treatment of epilepsy*, 3rd edn. Blackwell Publishing, Oxford.

Chapter 7

Epilepsy surgery

Key points

- *Epilepsy surgery* is defined as surgery carried out specifically to control epileptic seizures, and includes lesional surgery in which the primary indication is the control of seizures. It also implies a particular procedural approach to pre-surgical assessment.

- The pre-surgical assessment employs a different set of investigations to that used in other lesional surgery.

- The commonest operation carried out is the temporal lobectomy and vagus nerve stimulation.

- In well-selected patients, the temporal lobectomy will render up to 60% of patients seizure free in the long term. Adverse effects of the operation include risks of hemipareisis, memory disturbance, psychiatric and psychological change, and upper quadrantic visual field loss.

- Vagus nerve stimulation results in a 50% reduction in seizure frequency in approximately one-third of patients. Complications include infection, left vocal cord paralysis, cough, hoarseness, and cardiac conduction defects.

- Other operations include focal neocortical resections for other overt lesions ('lesionectomy'), non-lesional focal neocortical resections, hemispherectomy, and other multilobar resections, and functional procedures such as multiple subpial transection and corpus callosectomy.

- Various experimental procedures are under evaluation including focal radiation and deep-brain stimulation.

Epilepsy surgery is defined as surgery carried out specifically to control epileptic seizures. This includes operations on lesions such as tumours and vascular lesions where epilepsy is the primary indication for surgery. There is thus clearly an overlap with lesional surgery carried out for another primary reason (for instance, for oncological reasons, or vascular surgery to prevent haemorrhage, etc.). The latter operations are not usually considered as epilepsy surgery, even if the operation influences the epilepsy. The distinction though is not always clear-cut and the control of epilepsy can be an important additional consideration in the decision to undertake surgery in such cases. The term *epilepsy surgery* also implies a particular procedural approach to pre-surgical assessment and a different set of investigations to that usually employed in other lesional surgery. There are five main types of brain surgery carried out for epilepsy:

1. Temporal lobectomy for hippocampal sclerosis or other overt lesions in the mesial temporal lobe (approximately 65% of all epilepsy surgical operations)

2. Focal neocortical resections for overt lesions ('lesionectomy') (approximately 25% of all epilepsy surgical operations)

3. Non-lesional focal resections (approximately 5% of all epilepsy surgical operations)

4. Hemispherectomy, hemispherotomy, and other multilobar resections (approximately 4% of all epilepsy surgical operations)

5. Functional procedures—multiple subpial transection, corpus callosectomy, focal ablation, focal stimulation (approximately 1% of all epilepsy surgical operations)

Vagus nerve stimulation is another form of 'epilepsy surgery', which is not included in these figures but has become a relatively common type of surgical therapy for epilepsy.

As a general rule, epilepsy surgery should at least be considered in any patient with partial seizures that are intractable to drug therapy. The evaluation needs to be made by an experienced epilepsy surgery team, and will depend on the type of surgery being considered.

7.1 **Temporal lobectomy for hippocampal sclerosis or other lesions in the mesial temporal lobe**

Temporal lobectomy has been practiced widely since the 1950s. In those pre-imaging days, assessment was based on the clinical history and electroencephalogram (EEG). The advent of magnetic resonance imaging (MRI) has greatly improved the assessment process, as the lesion to be resected can, with MRI, be reliably visualized and quantified. The technique has evolved over the years, and, for hippocampal sclerosis, now involves a resection of the anterior portion of the temporal lobe to expose the hippocampus and then a resection of as much of the hippocampus and associated structures as possible. For resection of other lesions in the temporal lobe, the amount of hippocampal resection will vary according to the site of the lesion and the nature of the epilepsy. In spite of improvements in pre-surgical evaluation, the technique has not changed dramatically over the past half century, and there has been only a modest improvement in outcome due to better patient selection.

7.1.1 **Indications**

The usual indication is the presence of unilateral temporal lobe epilepsy in which the seizures are intractable to medical therapy. Intractability is of course difficult to define as it is essentially a retrospective concept. For pragmatic reasons, epilepsy is regarded as sufficiently intractable to contemplate surgery if it has been continuously active for 5yrs (or less in particularly severe epilepsy) in spite of adequate trials of therapy with five or more mainline antiepileptic drugs, and if seizures are frequent (more than one a month). A recent trend has been to define intractability earlier—after 2 or 3yrs of failure to respond to medical therapy. However, many patients who have had active epilepsy for 2–3yrs do respond to changing medical therapy later, and for this reason, 2–3yrs seems, to this author at least, generally too short a time to confirm an epilepsy as intractable.

The commonest underlying pathology is hippocampal sclerosis, although other temporal lobe lesions such as cavernomas and other vascular lesions, cortical dysplasia, and hamartomas and other tumours can also be resected via a temporal lobectomy.

7.1.2 **Pre-surgical assessment**

The purpose of pre-surgical assessment is shown in Table 7.1. All patients require (a) a detailed medical history; (b) appropriate interictal scalp EEG recording; (c) high-quality MRI at 1.5 or 3 Tesla with appropriate focus on the temporal lobe and including a T1, T2, and fluid attenuation inversion recovery (FLAIR) sequence and quantification of hippocampal volume and T2 measurement (see Figure 7.2); (d) a psychiatric assessment; (e) a neuropsychological assessment, focusing particularly on memory, language, and general ability. Most patients (over 90%) require an ictal EEG recording in addition, carried out via video-EEG telemetry. Selected patients (less than 10% of all) require intracranial EEG (see Figure 7.1), additional structure imaging, additional functional imaging with positron emission tomography (PET) or single photon emission tomography (SPECT) scanning, additional neurophysiological tests, sodium amytal test, or other neuropsychological tests. Examples of pre-surgical imaging studies are provided in Figures 7.1–7.3.

Table 7.1 Multifaceted nature of pre-surgical assessment for hippocampal epilepsy surgery

Medical history and ictal EEG	To confirm that the seizures are epileptic and to establish safety of surgery
Medical history	To confirm that the epilepsy is drug resistant
Medical history, ictal EEG, MRI, PET/SPECT, neuropsychological assessment, other techniques including MEG, fMRI	To identify the epileptogenic zone, to ensure it is unifocal
Neuropsychology	To assess risks to memory function and establish location of language function
Neuropsychiatric assessment	To assess risks of psychosis, depression, and other organic mental disorders after surgery
Medical consultation	To provide an assessment of risk vs. benefit of surgery for the patient to define outcome goals; define likely gains in quality of life; determine risks of surgical procedure — in terms of mortality, neurological morbidity, psychological, and social effects; counsel the patient, and ensure consent is informed

Figure 7.1 MRI showing position of depth electrodes implanted bilaterally in temporal lobes as part of a pre-surgical evaluation

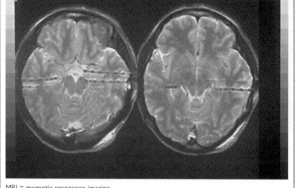

MRI = magnetic resonance imaging.

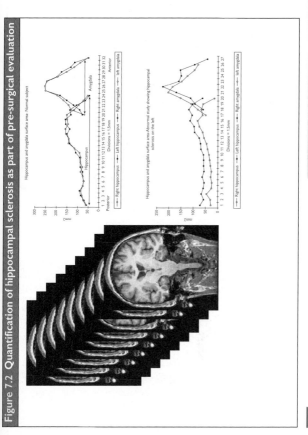

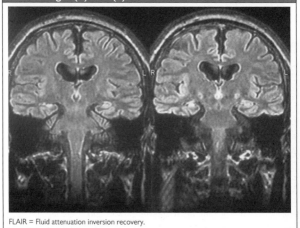

Figure 7.3 FLAIR sequence showing bilateral hippocampal sclerosis right (R)>left (L)

FLAIR = Fluid attenuation inversion recovery.

7.1.3 Pre-surgical counselling

Pre-surgical counselling is vital in all cases. The purpose is to explain the outcome of surgery, and to provide a detailed risk versus benefit analysis. It is important to ensure that the patient is fully informed and fully able to give informed consent.

7.1.4 'Red flags'

The following features point to a more guarded outcome, in particular to lowered rates of seizure freedom post-operatively:

- A history of generalized seizures. The outcome of temporal lobe surgery is best where the patient has a single type of complex partial seizure, without secondarily generalization.
- A normal MRI (i.e. showing no hippocampal abnormality)
- An MRI showing bilateral hippocampal changes or additional pathologies ('dual pathologies') (see Figure 7.3)
- A lack of concordance of MRI and EEG, where the EEG suggests a seizure onset in a location distant from the MRI abnormality.
- Ictal EEG which shows bilateral changes
- Discordant neuropsychological findings: the neuropsychological assessment suggests abnormalities outside the targeted hippocampal area.
- A post-encephalitic or post-traumatic aetiology for the hippocampal sclerosis (in contrast to those with hippocampal sclerosis associated with a history of febrile seizures or with no known cause).

- The presence of learning disability, in particular in patients with a very low IQ. These patients also may not be able to give informed consent for the operation.
- Age over 50yrs. The long-term results of surgery may be worse, due to lack of cerebral reserve.
- History of epileptic psychosis or other psychiatric disorder. The presence of an interictal psychosis is a contraindication to surgery. A history of severe psychiatric disorder needs careful assessment before surgery can be advised.

7.1.5 Outcome of temporal lobe resection

7.1.5.1 Seizure control

It is important to realize that temporal lobectomy does not guarantee long-term seizure control. At 1yr post-surgery, in published studies, overall 'seizure freedom' rates have generally ranged between 50% and 80% (median 70%), and at 5yrs, rates have ranged between 45% and 70%. 'Seizure freedom' in these studies includes patients who continue to have auras (or other 'non-disabling' seizures) or seizures occurring only on drug withdrawal, and the rates for true 'complete seizure freedom' are lower. Longer-term data are largely lacking, but one study has showed a 7% drop in seizure freedom rates from 5yrs to 10yrs after surgery (52% to 45%).

A further 10%–30% of patients, even if not completely seizure-free, achieve at least a 75% reduction of seizures in the year after surgery. Only 10%–20% of patients do not experience any improvement after surgery.

7.1.5.2 Immediate morbidity and mortality

Temporal lobectomy (Figure 7.4) has a number of potential complications (see Table 7.2). The commonest neurological deficits are as follows: superior quadrantanopia, due to damage to the optic radiation which loops through the posterior temporal lobe; hemiplegia due to damage to the anterior choroidal artery or pial vessels that lie on the surface of the midbrain mesial to the hippocampus; a permanent dysphasia in dominant hemisphere operations. Other risks of surgery include third nerve palsy, meningitis, bone or scalp infection, vascular spasm, subdural haematoma or empyema, hydrocephalus, and pneumocephalus. The overall risk of serious permanent neurological complications of temporal lobectomy in a modern experienced centre is in the order of 2%–3% (excluding psychiatric effects, cognitive effects and visual field loss), and the mortality rate of surgery is less than 0.5%.

7.1.5.3 Effects on memory

A profound amnesia occurs in less than 1% of cases, in modern practice. However, minor memory deficits are common and can be to some extent predicted by pre-operative neuropsychological testing—and this indeed is one major reason for carrying out the pre-operative assessment.

Figure 7.4 MRI scan after a left temporal lobectomy, showing extent of the mesial and lateral temporal lobe resection cavity

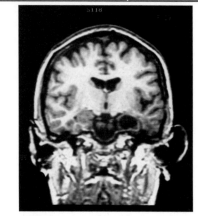

MRI = magnetic resonance imaging.

Table 7.2 Complications of temporal lobectomy

Complication	Rate (%)
Death	0.4
Transient hemiplegia	4
Permanent hemipareisis	2
Third nerve palsy	<1
Complete hemianopia	<2
Visual field loss	24
Depression[a]	34
Psychosis[a]	5
Global amnesia	<1
Significant memory loss	>10
Other cognitive effects	N/K
Other psychiatric effects	N/K

[a]In first year post-operation. (The rate of complications depends on the patients selection.) N/K = not known. Data taken from various sources—see Shorvon and Moran, 2009.

7.1.5.4 *Psychiatric and cognitive outcome*

The risk of psychosis or depression after temporal lobe surgery has been well studied, but other less obvious psychiatric morbidity less so. Post-operative psychosis occurs in approximately 5% of cases in the first year after surgery. A post-operative depressive illness occurs in up to 35% of patients in the first year after surgery. Less well studied are various behavioural changes which can also occur after temporal lobe surgery. These 'organic mental disorders' are generally mild and often undetected. They include changes in sexuality (hyposexual changes are more frequent than hypersexuality, but both occur), obsessional behaviour which can reach disabling levels, emotional blunting, asthenia, and other personality changes. Another risk is that of late deterioration due to lack of 'cerebral reserve' particularly in cases operated upon in mid- or late-adult life, but the extent of this risk is unclear.

7.1.5.5 *Psychosocial outcome*

After successful surgery, a readjustment to a life without epilepsy is needed. This can be difficult and there is often a sense of anti-climax, especially in the first 12 months following the operation. Moreover, if the operation fails, disappointment and depression are almost inevitable. Seizure freedom does not immediately reverse years of social isolation, a lack of self-confidence, and missed educational or career opportunities. Inter-personal relationships, which might have been based on dependency, can change, sometimes seemingly for the worse. A post-operative counselling and rehabilitation programme can be helpful. Overall though, when seizure freedom is obtained, and where patients have been carefully selected, the temporal lobectomy can have an extraordinarily positive effect, allowing a person to engage in all aspects of life with confidence and unencumbered by the constant fear and undermining influence of seizures.

7.2 Focal resections for other overt lesions ('lesionectomy')

The widespread use of MRI has demonstrated that there are often small structural lesions causing focal epilepsy in temporal neocortex or extratemporal regions. These may be susceptible to resective surgery in an attempt to control epilepsy. The commonest such lesions are small slow-growing or benign tumours, small arteriovenous malformations (AVMs) and cavernomas, but other larger AVMs, malformations of cortical development, post-traumatic and post-infective damage can also be resected. The general principles of surgery and the investigatory approach are broadly similar to that of mesial temporal epilepsy. However, there are important differences in emphasis. The three key determinants of surgical outcome are the aetiology of the lesion, the extent of the resection, and the site of the resection.

The pre-surgical assessment focuses on determining aetiology, the extent of the lesion, the extent of epileptogenic areas in the brain, and the risk of resection. There is often a need for extensive EEG, including depth EEG, and sophisticated structural imaging and functional imaging techniques, including sometimes PET and SPECT scanning.

The lesions with the best outcome following lesionectomy are cavernomas and small benign tumours, provided that the lesion can be completely removed and that there is no concomitant pathology. Thus, patients with hamartomas and other benign tumours, low grade gliomas, dysembryoplastic neuro-epithelial tumours, and cavernomas, have a 50%–80% chance of seizure freedom following removal of the lesion. In situations where the lesion is less well defined or is associated with more widespread abnormalities, the potential for seizure control is reduced; for instance, in patients with cortical dysplasia, where epileptogenic abnormalities are widespread often beyond the structural abnormalities visible on the MRI scan. Temporal lobe lesions are frequently associated with hippocampal sclerosis, and experience dictates that removal of both the lesion and the hippocampus is often necessary for a successful outcome. The complications of surgery depend on the location of the lesion, and in particular its proximity to eloquent cortex. Resections in the frontal lobe are generally less successful than temporal lobe surgery, with approximately 30%–40% become seizure free.

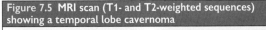

Figure 7.5 MRI scan (T1- and T2-weighted sequences) showing a temporal lobe cavernoma

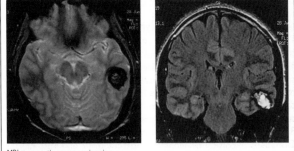

MRI = magnetic resonance imaging.

7.3 **Non-lesional focal resections**

MRI has been of great benefit to the assessment of patients for epilepsy surgery. Its excellent sensitivity can demonstrate even small structural lesions, which are the surgical targets. Where routine MRI is normal, MRI using sophisticated 'epilepsy protocols' will often reveal small lesions not previously suspected. This is especially the case in patients with small vascular lesions or tumours or cortical dysplasia. MRI scanning should be tailored to the individual problem (for instance, with special hippocampal views or cortical reformatting). In a few cases though of severe, medically intractable focal epilepsy, the MRI is normal even after the application of advanced techniques. In these 'non-lesional' or 'MRI-negative' cases, the localization of the epileptogenic zone depends largely on clinical and EEG evaluation, and functional imaging. The principles of surgical evaluation are essentially the same as in lesion cases—and are directed at determining the site and extent of the epileptogenic zone and the risks of resective surgery of this zone. Invasive EEG is often required as is PET or SPECT scanning or other functional MRI techniques.

The outcome in MRI negative cases is generally less good, and surgery should be considered only after careful evaluation. In general terms, the bigger the resection, the better is the outcome. In young children particularly, large resections carry less functional penalty as brain plasticity allows reallocation of function during subsequent development, and thus in infants with devastating epilepsy, large-scale resections, for instance, guided by interictal PET hypoperfusion, are considered appropriate even where no lesion and no focal EEG disturbance is present. In adults with normal MRI large cortical resections (for instance, a frontal lobectomy for epilepsy originating in anterior frontal regions) result in a seizure-free rate of less than 30%.

7.5 **Hemispherectomy**

This term covers a variety of operative techniques in which large parts of one cerebral hemisphere are excised and in which the two cerebral hemispheres are disconnected from the other. These are operations carried out in children or adolescents (and occasionally adults) with medically refractory seizures due to severe unilateral hemisphere damage—the common pathologies are perinatal stroke, hemimegencephaly or other major congenital disorder, Sturge–Weber syndromes, Rasmussen's encephalitis, or other post-natal unihemispheric injury. Only patients with severe epilepsy should be considered for this operation, with usually multiple seizure types and frequent (>5) daily seizures. The great majority of suitable candidates for hemispherectomy also have a pre-operative severe fixed hemiparesis, as a result of the hemispheric damage, sometimes associated with other signs, such as hemianopia or hemisensory loss. The operation is restricted to those in which the hemiparesis is severe enough to impair the performance of individual finger movements. If the operation is performed on the language dominant hemisphere, permanent aphasia will result unless language functions can be transferred to the other hemisphere by cortical plasticity. For this reason, it is possible to carry out dominant hemispherectomy before the age of 5 without any impairment of language functions. However, the operation should generally not be carried out in a dominant hemisphere after the age of 9yrs. Preoperative assessment includes EEG and neuroimaging.

The original surgical operation, the *anatomical hemispherectomy*, has been now largely been abandoned because of late post-operative complications (notably superficial cerebral haemosiderosis and of late hydrocephalus). Various alternatives have been devised, and the most widely used is the *Functional Hemispherectomy* which consists of a subtotal anatomical hemispherectomy with complete physiological disconnection.

The outcome of hemispherectomy in carefully selected patients is excellent. Complete seizure control is expected in approximately 70%–80%, and ≥80% improvement in seizures in 90%–95% of suitably selected and competently operated cases. Secondary gains in terms of behaviour and psychosocial development usually also occur. Some children will develop to the stage where independent living and work are possible.

7.6 Corpus callosotomy (corpus callosectomy)

This operation involves the functional disconnection of the two cerebral hemispheres by transection of the corpus callosum. It has a desynchronizing effect on epileptic activity, and can inhibit seizures, although exactly how or why is unclear. The operation is now primarily reserved for patients with severe secondarily generalized epilepsy manifest by frequent drop attacks causing injury, in whom medical therapy is ineffective and in whom other surgical procedures are not possible. Many of these patients have the *Lennox–Gastaut syndrome*. It can also be used in combination with resective surgery, and especially after frontal lobe trauma or abscess. Pre-surgical evaluation includes EEG, MRI, and psychometric assessment. Patients with preoperative EEG showing bilateral synchronous epileptic discharges or lateralized abnormalities tend to have a better outcome than those with multifocal EEG discharges.

The operation must be considered a palliative procedure, intended to reduce seizure severity and in particular to reduce injuries due to falls. Short-term seizure freedom does occur in approximately 5%–10% of cases but there is a strong tendency for seizures to relapse over months or years, and no patient should undergo this operation in the expectation of full seizure control. Various complications can occur including hemipareisis, a very characteristic transient disconnection syndrome with mutism, urinary incontinence, and bilateral leg weakness. A posterior disconnection syndrome can occur, and most patients will exhibit elements of a 'split brain' profile on neuropsychological testing although this causes remarkably little disability in everyday living. Overall, the risks of permanent severe deficits after corpus callosal section, either neurological or neuropsychological, are of the order of 5%–10%, and there is a mortality rate of approximately 1%–5%. The operation is now performed far less often than in the past, largely because of the introduction of vagus nerve stimulation.

7.7 Multiple subpial transaction

In this operation, parallel rows of 4–5mm deep cortical incisions are ploughed perpendicular to the cortical surface. This is done on the theoretical basis that the transections sever horizontal cortical connections and thus disrupt the lateral recruitment of neurones, which is essential in producing synchronized epileptic discharges. At the same time, normal function is preserved as this is supported largely by vertically oriented afferent and efferent connections. The procedure is usually performed where the epileptogenic zone involves eloquent brain cortex, in which resection would result in significant neurological deficit. It has thus been principally applied to patients with epileptic foci in language, or primary sensory or motor cortex. In many cases, it has been combined with a lesion resection when the lesion is in or adjacent to eloquent cortex.

The outcome is dependent on the underlying pathology and the surgical technique. Generally, a marked reduction in seizures occurs in the short term in 60%–80% of patients, but the longer-term outcome is not as good. Neurological deficits occurred post-operatively in approximately 20% of patients. It is an operation restricted to a small number of patients and should be carried out only in units with special expertise.

7.8 Brain stimulation

This is an essentially experimental technique at present. Deep brain stimulation (DBS) has become possible because of the improved MRI, better surgical instrumentation, and stimulation technology. The favoured targets include caudate nucleus, centromedian nucleus of the thalamus, anterior thalamic nucleus, and subthalamic nucleus. Direct stimulation of the epileptic focus, in both the neocortex and the hippocampus, has also been attempted. A recent technology has been developed that switches on stimulation at the beginning of a seizure recorded on EEG via intracranial electrodes. The efficacy of these techniques is under current investigation.

7.9 **Gamma knife/proton beam 'surgery'**

It is possible, using a 'gamma knife' or other technologies to focus radiation on to small target areas of brain, with a view to achieving focal ablation of brain tissue. This is quite widely used in epilepsy surgery for small vascular lesions, such as cavernomas, and for surgical targets, such as hypothalamic hamartomas, where resection carries particular risk. Focused radiation carries the risk of late-occurring brain necrosis and other complications. It is also under trial for hippocampal sclerosis, but the relative benefits and risks compared to resective surgery for hippocampal sclerosis have not been fully established.

7.10 **Vagus nerve stimulation**

This operation has been approved by the regulatory authorities for approximately 10yrs. It is a palliative procedure and now used widely throughout the world. The operation comprises the implantation of a stimulator below the skin in the chest wall with bipolar electrodes wrapped around the left vagus nerve. The vagus nerve is then stimulated with the programme of stimulation (strength of current, duration of stimulation, and pattern of stimulation pulses) tailored for the individual. It is a relatively minor procedure, lacking the inherent risks of intracranial surgery, and hence its immediate attraction to physicians and patients alike.

The effectiveness and safety of vagus nerve stimulation were investigated in blinded and randomized clinical trials in a manner identical to that applied to new antiepileptic drugs. Approximately one-third of patients in these trials experienced a 50% reduction in seizure frequency. Virtually no patient is rendered seizure free by the procedure.

There are a number of potential peri-operative complications including infection, left vocal cord paralysis, and lower facial muscle paresis. Dyspnoea, cough, and hoarseness are not uncommon during stimulation. Cardiac conduction defects can occur.

The indications for the procedure are not fully explored, but currently it is used in patients who have failed to respond to conventional medical therapy, and in whom resective surgical therapy is not appropriate, or in whom corpus callosotomy would be considered. There is no clear evidence that one seizure type does better than any other. Its main advantage is that it does not have the cognitive and CNS side effects associated with conventional antiepileptic medication. The procedure has not, in the opinion of many, lived up to the promise apparent from the clinical trials. Few, if any, patients have gained seizure freedom from the technique, and there appears often to be little or no effect at all.

References and further reading

Arzimanoglou A, Guerrini R, and Aicardi J (2003). *Aicardi's epilepsy in children*, 3rd edn. Lippincott, Williams and Wilkins, Philadelphia.

Bien CG, Kurthen M, Baron K, *et al.* (2001). Long-term seizure outcome and antiepileptic drug treatment in surgically treated temporal lobe epilepsy patients: a controlled study. *Epilepsia*, **42**, 1416–21.

Engel J Jr (ed.) (1993). *Surgical treatment of the epilepsies*, 2nd edn. Raven Press, New York.

Engel J Jr and Pedley TA (eds) (2008). *Epilepsy: a comprehensive textbook*, 2nd edn. Lippincott-Raven, Philadelphia.

ILAE Commission Report (1997). Recommendations for Neuroimaging of Patients with Epilepsy. Commission on Neuroimaging of the International League Against Epilepsy. *Epilepsia*, **38**, 1255–6.

ILAE Commission Report (1998). Guidelines for Neuroimaging Evaluation of Patients with Uncontrolled Epilepsy Considered for Surgery. Commission on Neuroimaging of the International League Against Epilepsy. *Epilepsia*, **39**, 1375–6.

ILAE Commission Report (2000). Commission on Diagnostic Strategies. Recommendations for Functional Neuroimaging of Persons with Epilepsy. Neuroimaging Subcommission of the International League Against Epilepsy. *Epilepsia*, **41**, 1350–6.

Jarrar RG, Buchhalter JR, Meyer FB, Sharbrough FW, and Laws E (2002). Long-term follow-up of temporal lobectomy in children. *Neurology*, **59**, 1635–7.

Lüders HO (eds) (2008) *Textbook of epilepsy surgery*. Informa, London.

Luders H and Comair Y (eds) (2001). *Epilepsy surgery*, 2nd edn. Lippincott, Williams and Wilkins, Philadelphia.

Mathern GW (ed) (1999). Pediatric epilepsy and epilepsy surgery. *Developmental Neuroscience*, **21**, 159–408.

Mauguiere F and Ryvlin P (2004). The role of PET in presurgical assessment of partial epilepsies. *Epileptic Disorders*, **6**, 193–215.

McIntosh AM, Kalnins RM, Mitchell LA, Fabinyi GC, Briellmann RS, and Berkovic SF (2004). Temporal lobectomy: long-term seizure outcome, late recurrence and risks for seizure recurrence. *Brain,* **27**, 2018–30.

Miller JW and Silbergeld DL (eds) (2006). *Epilepsy surgery: principles and controversies*. Taylor & Francis, New York.

Moran N, Shorvon SD (2009). The surgery of temporal lobe epilepsy 11-surgical complications and long-term adverse effects. In Shorvon SD, Pedley TA (eds). *The Epilepsies 3*, Vol 33, (p. 307–21), Blue book of Neurology series. Saunders, Philadelphia.

Polkey CE (2004). Clinical outcome of epilepsy surgery. *Current Opinion in Neurology*, **17**, 173–8.

Porter BE, Judkins AR, Clancy RR, Duhaime A, Dlugos DJ, and Golden JA (2003). Dysplasia: a common finding in intractable pediatric temporal lobe epilepsy. *Neurology*, **61**, 365–8.

Shorvon SD (2005). *Handbook of epilepsy treatment: forms, causes and therapy in children and adults*. Blackwell Science, Oxford.

Shorvon SD, Pedley TA (eds) (2009). *The Epilepsies 3*, vol 33, Blue book of Neurology series. Saunders, Philadelphia.

Shorvon SD, Perucca E, Engel J (eds) (2009). *The treatment of epilepsy*, 3rd edn. Blackwell Publishing, Oxford.

Sperling MR, Walczak TS, Berg AT, Shinnar S, Pacia S. (2004). Mortality after surgical or medical therapy for refractory epilepsy. *Epilepsia*, **45**(Suppl 7), 190–1.

Vickrey B, Hays R, Engel J, Bazil C. (1995). Outcome assessment for epilepsy surgery: the impact of measuring health-related quality of life. *Annals of Neurology*, **37**, 158–166.

Wheless JW and Baumgartner J (2004). Vagus nerve stimulation therapy. *Drugs Today (Barc)*, **40**, 501–15.

Wiebe S, Blume WT, Girvin JP, and Eliasziw M (2001). A randomized, controlled trial of surgery for temporal lobe epilepsy. *The New England Journal of Medicine*, **345**, 311–18.

Wieser HG and Elger CE (eds) (1987). *Presurgical evaluation of epileptics: basics, techniques, implications*. Springer-Verlag, Berlin.

Wieser HG, Blume WT, Fish D, Vickrey B, Spencer S, Langfitt JT (2001). Proposal for a new classification of outcome with respect to epileptic seizures following epilepsy surgery. Commission on Neurosurgery of the International League Against Epilepsy (ILAE) 1997–2001. *Epilepsia*, **42**, 282–6.

Zentner J and Seeger W (eds) (2003). *Surgical treatment of epilepsy*. Springer-Verlag, New York.

Chapter 8

Emergency treatment of epileptic seizures

Key points

- Most seizures are self-terminating and require no emergency drug therapy.
- Simple first aid measures are helpful at the time of a seizure.
- Many patients have clusters of seizures and in this situation emergency drug therapy with benzodiazepines can be given to prevent recurrence. Similarly oral benzodiazepine therapy can be given on an occasional basis, as one-off prophylaxis, to prevent a seizure.
- Status epilepticus is defined as a condition in which epileptic seizures continue, or are repeated without recovery, for a period of 30min or more. It can take many forms.
- Tonic-clonic status epilepticus is a medical emergency requiring immediate therapy. A strict treatment protocol should be followed and this improves outcome.
- Other forms of status epilepticus also require specific treatment.

Most seizures are self-terminating and require no emergency treatment. Simple first aid measures during and after the seizure can be taken but little else is needed. Emergency antiepileptic therapy is needed in prolonged seizures, is sometimes helpful in preventing serial seizures and is mandatory in status epilepticus. These topics are considered in turn in this chapter.

8.1 First aid measures

Advise on first aid measures should be given to all patients and their carers. If a seizure is likely to occur in any particular situation, for instance, at school or at work, it is often also useful to provide simple first aid advice to those who might be present. Such information will lessen the impact of a sudden epileptic seizure, which can be frightening and disturbing to onlookers, and reduce embarrassment to the sufferer.

8.1.1 **Tonic-clonic seizures**

No medication is needed, or indeed would have any point, during or after most short-lived tonic-clonic seizures. However, first aid measures can be very useful. During the seizure, the patient should be moved into a position of safety. The head should be protected and tight neckware released. Measures should be taken to avoid injury (e.g. from hot radiators, fire, top of stairs, water, road traffic). No attempt should be made to open the mouth or force anything between the teeth. The individual should be placed lying down in the recovery position as soon as possible.

It is essential to check that the airway is not obstructed and that the pulse is adequate, during the seizure and in its immediate aftermath. Sometimes, breathing ceases in a seizure and resumption of respiration can be triggered by physical (touching or shaking) or verbal stimulation. Assistance should be sought if there is any concern over cardiac function.

After a seizure, a check should be made to ensure that there are no injuries.

As recovery occurs, the individual should be comforted and reassured. It is important to stay in attendance until full consciousness has returned and confusion has faded. An ambulance should not generally be called in a person with known epilepsy if seizures are occurring regularly and the attack subsides quickly and is uneventful (Box 8.1).

Box 8.1 When to call an ambulance because of an epileptic seizure

- All patients in whom there is no known history of epilepsy or epileptic seizures (if in doubt, call an ambulance).
- In patients with known active epilepsy, an ambulance is required after a seizure only if
  - Injury has occurred
  - Convulsive movements continue for longer than 10min (or longer than is customary for the individual patient)
  - Consciousness is not rapidly regained
  - Seizures rapidly recur
  - Cardiorespiratory function is impaired
  - Seizure has new clinical features (not customary for the individual patient)

8.1.2 Nonconvulsive seizures

Again, drug treatment is neither indicated nor desirable in short attacks. The main emphasis should be on minimizing risk. If confusion is present, it may be necessary to take measures to prevent injury or danger, for instance, from wandering about. In doing so, forcible restraint should be kept to a minimum, as this can increase confusion and cause agitation or occasional violence.

8.2 Serial seizures and one-off prophylaxis

In a proportion of patients, seizures tend to occur in clusters. This is a particularly common pattern in partial seizures in temporal or frontal lobe epilepsy where a cluster can last for hours or several days, or in epilepsy with generalized absence seizures or myoclonus, where a cluster may continue for minutes or hours. In other patients, there is a tendency for a first convulsion to be followed by a second convulsion (and sometimes a further series) in the minutes or hours after a first attack. Sometimes, serial seizures are a warning of impending status epilepticus. In all these situations, the administration of emergency medication after the early seizures can prevent recurrence (Table 8.1).

The choice of medication depends on the expected timing of the recurrence. If recurrence is expected over hours, an oral benzodiazepine is often given. The usual choice is a single dose of clobazam. This will take 60min or so to take effect and last for 12–24hr. If the recurrence is expected more quickly, parenteral benzodiazepine therapy is needed. In out of the hospital settings, this is usually administered as rectal diazepam or buccal midazolam. Rectal diazepam is effective usually within 10–20min and the effects persist for 4hr. It is safe and easy to administer, although often embarrassing for the sufferer. Buccal midazolam is increasingly used as an alternative and is preferred by patients and carers for ease of use and preservation

Table 8.1 Antiepileptic drugs used to prevent serial seizures			
Drug	Route of administration	Adult dose	Paediatric dose
Clobazam	Oral	10–20mg	
Diazepam	Oral	10–20mg	0.25–0.5mg/kg
	Rectal administration	10–30mg	0.5–0.75mg/kg
Midazolam	Buccal/IM (unlicensed indications)	10mg	6–12 months: 2.5mg 1–5yrs: 5mg 5–10>yrs: 7.5mg
Paraldehyde	Rectal	5–10mL	0.1–0.35mL/kg

of dignity (however the product is currently only available as an unlicensed product). Midazolam is instilled into the mouth where it is rapidly absorbed through the buccal mucosa. It takes effect within 5–10min and the effects persist for several hours. Midazolam can alternatively be given by intranasal or intramuscular (IM) injection (unlicensed use). Rectal paraldehyde is still occasionally used as an alternative, especially in children.

If the patient is in a hospital setting, it is usual to give intravenous (IV) benzodiazepines, which are quicker and more effective. The choice is usually between diazepam or lorazepam (unlicensed use).

The parenteral administration of any benzodiazepine in a small proportion of cases will cause severe respiratory depression, and the patient should never be left unattended after administration until full recovery has occurred. All the benzodiazepines (and especially midazolam) can cause drowsiness or sleep at these doses.

Clobazam (10mg) can be given as a single dose as one-off prophylaxis on occasions where a seizure needs to be particularly avoided (e.g. travel, exams, public ceremony, etc.). It is often very effective used in this way.

8.3 Tonic-clonic status epilepticus

Tonic-clonic status epilepticus is a medical emergency. Hospitalization is required and therapy should be instituted as quickly as possible to prevent cerebral damage. The mortality rate of established tonic-clonic status epilepticus is approximately 20%, and the rates of morbidity and mortality increase the longer the seizure activity is allowed to continue.

Sixty per cent of cases of status epilepticus occur out of the blue, in patients without a history of epilepsy and in the context of acute brain injury, for instance, due to a stroke, encephalitis, trauma, metabolic disturbance, or toxin exposure. In these situations, usually nothing can be done to prevent the occurrence of the status epilepticus. In the other 40%, the status epilepticus occurs in the context of existing epilepsy, and in such cases there is often a warning (premonitory) period before the episode of status is initiated during which time, emergency therapy will prevent the status developing.

8.3.1 Establish aetiology

It is vital in all cases of status epilepticus to establish the cause. The range of causes differs with age and also depends on whether the patient has a history of established epilepsy. The investigations required vary in different clinical circumstances. Computer tomography (CT) or magnetic resonance imaging (MRI) and cerebrospinal fluid examination are often necessary and should be carried out as soon as the emergency measures have stabilized the patient's clinical state and antiepileptic drug therapy has been initiated. Lumber puncture should be undertaken only with facilities for resuscitation available as intracranial pressure is often elevated in status epilepticus.

In *de novo* status epilepticus, there is almost always an acute cerebral disturbance—and common causes are encephalitis, meningitis, trauma, stroke, acute toxin ingestion, fever, and acute metabolic or immunological disturbance. In patients with known epilepsy, the status epilepticus is usually caused by antiepileptic drug withdrawal or reduction, or an acute intercurrent illness. If the status epilepticus has been precipitated by drug withdrawal, the immediate restitution of the withdrawn drug, even at lower doses, will usually rapidly terminate the status epilepticus.

8.3.2 **Drug treatment of tonic-clonic status epilepticus**
The drug treatment of tonic-clonic status epilepticus should be staged. A systematic protocol-driven approach is important in this emergency situation and the simple application of a written protocol in an A&E department has been shown to improve prognosis.

8.3.2.1 *Stage of premonitory status epilepticus*
In patients with existing epilepsy, the episode of status is often heralded by a period of increasing seizure activity ('the stage of premonitory status epilepticus'). The seizures may take the form of recurrent absence seizures or myoclonus, causing mild obtundation or confusion (in Idiopathic Generalized Epilepsy) or recurrent focal seizures (in partial epilepsy). These can increase in frequency or severity, and this period may last minutes or hours. This pattern, and the fact that it indicates impending status, is often easily recognized by the individual or carers. In this situation, parenteral benzodiazepine drugs can be given to prevent the status (see Tables 8.1 and 8.2). The drug administration can be repeated once after 10min if initially ineffective.

8.3.2.2 *Stage of early status epilepticus*
This is defined as the first 30min of the episode of status epilepticus (continuous or rapidly recurring tonic-clonic seizures). Therapy is with IV benzodiazepine drugs. The usual choice is IV lorazepam, diazepam, or clonazepam (Table 8.2). If benzodiazepines have already been given (in either serial seizures or in the premonitory stage), this stage is omitted and therapy pursued as described below.

8.3.2.3 *Stage of established status epilepticus*
This is defined as the period between 30min and 60/90min of status epilepticus, if early-stage treatment has failed. The traditional therapy is with IV phenytoin or phenobarbital, although increasingly IV valproate and levetiracetam are now given (albeit off label and without supporting trial data) (Table 8.3). The risk of complications and long-term morbidity are greater in this stage, and the patient may need ITU care.

Table 8.2 Antiepileptic drugs used in the early stages

Drug	Route of administration	Adult dose	Paediatric dose
Diazepam	IV bolus (not exceeding 2–5mg/min)	10–20mg	0.25–0.5mg/kg
	Rectal administration	10–30mg	Neonate: 1.25–2.5mg Child 1 month–2yrs: 5mg 2–12yrs: 5–10mg 12–18yrs: 10mg
Clonazepam	IV bolus	1mg	0.5mg
Lorazepam	IV bolus	0.07mg/kg (usually 4mg)	0.1mg/kg

Table 8.3 Antiepileptic drugs used in the stage of established status epilepticus

Drug	Route of administration	Adult dose	Paediatric dose
Fosphenytoin	IV bolus (not exceeding 100mg PE/min)	15–20mg PE/kg	
Levetiracetam[a]	IV	1000–4000mg	N/A
Phenytoin	IV bolus/infusion (not exceeding 50mg/min)	15–20mg/kg	20mg/kg at 1–3/kg/min
Phenobarbital	IV bolus (not exceeding 100mg/min)	10–20mg/kg (max. 1g)	15–20mg/kg
Valproate[a]	IV bolus	10mg/kg	20–40mg/kg

[a]These are off-label indications, and not supported by any randomized clinical trials, but are nevertheless widely used.
PE = phenytoin equivalents.

8.3.2.4 *Stage of refractory status epilepticus*

This stage is reached if treatment of the earlier stages has been given and has failed, and the status has continued for over 60–120min. At this point, general anaesthesia is advised. Full intensive monitoring is required, including intra-arterial blood pressure, oximetry, and sometimes central venous and pulmonary artery pressure monitoring. The choice of anaesthetic is usually made by the anaesthetists in charge of ITU, and commonly midazolam, propofol, or thiopental/pentobarbital is given (Table 8.4). There are no comparative trials and the choice is essentially arbitrary. Anaesthesia should be maintained ideally at a level which produces the burst suppression pattern on the electro-encephalogram (EEG), with inter-burst intervals of between 2sec and 30sec, although often this depth of anaesthesia is not possible, and the anaesthetic dosage is limited by hypotension.

Table 8.4 Anaesthetic drugs used in the stage of refractory status epilepticus

Drug	Dose
Midazolam	0.1–0.3mg/kg at 4mg/min bolus followed by infusion at 0.05–0.4mg/kg/hr
Thiopental	100–250mg bolus over 20sec then further 50mg boluses every 2–3min until seizures are controlled; then infusion to maintain burst suppression (3–5mg/kg/hr). Child 1 month–18yrs: initially up to 4mg/kg by slow intravenous injection, then up to 8mg/kg/hr by continuous intravenous infusion
Pentobarbital	10–20mg/kg at 25mg/min then 0.5–1mg/kg/hr increasing to 1–3mg/kg/hr
Propofol	2mg/kg then 5–10mg/kg/hr

When seizures have been controlled for 12hr, the drug dosage should be slowly reduced over a further 12hrs. If seizures recur, the anaesthetic agent should be given again for another 12hr, and then withdrawal be attempted again. This cycle may need to be repeated every 24–48hr until seizure control is achieved. In occasional cases, anaesthesia thus given may be needed for weeks.

8.3.3 General measures

In addition to drug therapy, the management of tonic-clonic status epilepticus requires attention to the following aspects:

8.3.3.1 *Cardiorespiratory resuscitation*

As soon as a patient presents in status, it is essential to assess cardio-respiratory function, to secure the airway, and to resuscitate where necessary. Oxygen should always be administered, as hypoxia is often unexpectedly severe.

8.3.3.2 *Monitor neurological status, vital signs, and laboratory tests*

Regular neurological observations and measurements of pulse, blood pressure, and temperature should be initiated. Electrocardiogram (ECG), biochemical, blood gas, pH, clotting, and haematological measures should be monitored.

8.3.3.3 *Intravenous lines*

Fluid replacement is often required, preferably with 0.9% sodium chloride (normal or physiological saline) rather than 5% glucose solutions. Drug administration requires IV access. If two antiepileptic drugs are needed, for example, phenytoin and diazepam, two IV lines should be sited. The lines should be in large veins, as many antiepileptic drugs cause phlebitis and thrombosis at the site of infusion. Arterial lines must never be used for administering drugs.

8.3.3.4 *Emergency investigations*

Blood should be drawn, immediately on presentation, for the emergency measurement of blood gases, sugar, renal and liver function, calcium and magnesium levels, full haematological screen (including platelets), blood clotting measures, and anti-convulsant levels. Serum (50mL) should also be saved for future analysis if the cause of the status epilepticus is uncertain. Other investigations depend on the clinical circumstances.

8.3.3.5 *Intravenous glucose, thiamine, magnesium, pyridoxine*

Fifty per cent glucose solution (50mL) IV should be given urgently if hypoglycaemia is suspected. Routine glucose administration in non-hypoglycaemic patients should be avoided as there is some evidence that this can aggravate neuronal damage.

If there is a history of alcoholism, or other compromised nutritional states, 250mg of thiamine (e.g. as the high-potency IV formulation of Pabrinex®, 10mL of which contains 250mg) should also be given slowly (infused over 10min). If glucose is given in alcoholics without thiamine, neuronal damage can be exacerbated.

IV magnesium (2–4g magnesium sulfate over 20min) is often given, even if there is no evidence of deficiency. Occult pyridoxine deficiency can present as status epilepticus, and IV pyridoxine should also be given to children under the age of 3yrs, who have a prior history of epilepsy, and to all neonates. It is often given as a precautionary measure to all children and adults in prolonged status.

8.3.3.6 *Acidosis*

Occasionally, the administration of bicarbonate acidosis is needed to correct acidosis. This should not be routinely given and usually acidosis is better and rapidly corrected by controlling respiration and abolishing seizure motor activity.

8.3.3.7 *Pressor therapy*

Prolonged status epilepticus can result in hypotension, and this tendency is exacerbated by IV drug therapy. Pressor therapy is therefore often required. Dopamine is used at a dose titrated to the desired haemodynamic and renal responses (usually initially between 2 and 5mcg/kg/min, but this can be increased to over 20mcg/kg/min in severe hypotension). ECG monitoring is required, as conduction defects may occur, and particular care is needed in dosing in the presence of cardiac failure.

8.3.3.8 *Long-term anti-convulsant therapy*

In tandem with emergency treatment, it is also vital to initiate the maintenance of antiepileptic therapy, via a nasogastric tube to provide long-term control when the emergency therapy is withdrawn. The choice of drug depends on previous therapy, the type of epilepsy, and the clinical setting. If phenytoin or phenobarbital have been used as emergency treatment, maintenance doses can be continued orally (through a nasogastric tube) guided by serum level monitoring.

8.3.3.9 *Cerebral oedema and raised intracranial pressure*

If cerebral oedema develops or if intracranial pressure is high, this can be controlled usually by intermittent positive pressure ventilation or high-dose corticosteroid therapy (4mg dexamethasone every 6hr). Mannitol infusion is usually given only as an emergency respite in incipient tentorial coning. Neurosurgical decompression is occasionally required. Continuous intracranial pressure monitoring is sometimes needed, especially in children, if the episode of status is prolonged.

8.3.3.10 *Seizure and EEG monitoring*

In comatose ventilated patients, motor activity can be barely visible even if the electrographic seizure activity persists. Continuous or regularly repeated EEG monitoring is necessary in this situation to assess the effectiveness of antiepileptic therapy and the depth of anaesthesia.

8.3.3.11 *Cardiac arrhythmia*

Cardiac arrhythmias pose a substantial risk in severe status, caused by autonomic hyperactivity, metabolic derangement, and the infusion of high-dose antiepileptic and anaesthetic drugs. Continuous ECG monitoring is mandatory, and arrhythmias are treated in the conventional manner.

8.3.3.12 *Preventing other medical complications*

Acute renal impairment can be due to myoglobinuria, disseminated intravascular coagulation, hypotension, and hypoxia. Acute hepatic failure can also have various causes, including hypersensitivity reactions to administered drugs. Some of the complications encountered in tonic-clonic status are listed in Table 8.5. These often need emergency treatment in their own right. Failure to do so can perpetuate the status and worsen outcome.

Table 8.5 Some medical complications of tonic-clonic status epilepticus

Cerebral	Hypoxia, cerebral oedema, ↑ICP, cerebral vein/sinus thrombosis, cerebral haemorrhage, excitotoxic brain injury
Cardiorespiratory	Hypotension, cardiac failure, arrhythmia, embolism, cardiogenic shock, respiratory failure, pulmonary oedema and hypertension, and aspiration
Autonomic and metabolic	Hyperpyrexia, sweating, hypersecretion, shock, dehydration, electrolyte imbalance, acute renal failure, acute hepatic failure
Other medical	DIC, rhabdomyolysis, pancreatic failure, infection, fractures, thrombophlebitis, dermal injury, venous thrombosis

DIC = disseminated intravascular coagulation; ICP = intracranial pressure.

8.4 **Other forms of status epilepticus**

There are many other forms of status epilepticus. Most are nonconvulsive forms and most do not generally require IV or ITU therapy.

8.4.1 **Complex partial status epilepticus**

Episodes of complex partial status are not uncommon in patients with focal epilepsy, and are often self-limiting. A fluctuating or continuous confusional state is the usual leading clinical feature. This can vary from profound stupor with little response to external stimuli in some cases, to others in whom subtle abnormalities on cognitive testing are the only signs. Amnesia, behavioural changes, speech and language disturbance, and motor and autonomic features are common features. Periods of complex partial status usually last for several hours but on occasions persist for days or even weeks. Complex partial status can also follow a secondary generalized tonic-clonic seizure (or cluster of seizures). Episodes are often recurrent. The prognosis is generally good, and it is rare for the episodes to be life-threatening or to cause significant cerebral damage. The condition often remits spontaneously, but if treatment is needed, oral benzodiazepines (diazepam or clobazam) are usually given as first-line therapy. If further therapy is needed, oral or IV phenytoin; phenobarbital or valproate; or other oral or IV antiepileptic drugs can be given. Usually non-ITU therapy suffices, but in occasional patients in whom the status is persistent and life-threatening, a protocol similar to that of the treatment of tonic-clonic status epilepticus will be needed.

8.4.2 **Absence status epilepticus**

This form of status epilepticus occurs only in patients with absence epilepsy. It is usually rapidly terminated by benzodiazepine therapy given as IV bolus doses. The usual drugs are as follows: diazepam 0.2–0.3mg/kg, clonazepam 1mg (0.25–0.5mg in children), or lorazepam 0.07mg/kg (0.1mg/kg in children). The bolus doses can be repeated if required. If this is ineffective, IV valproate or levetiracetam can be given.

8.4.3 **Atypical absence status**

This form of status is common in patients with diffuse cerebral damage and typically seen as part of the *Lennox–Gastaut syndrome*. In contrast to *typical absence status epilepticus*, this condition is usually poorly responsive to IV benzodiazepines, which should, in any case, be given cautiously, as they can induce tonic status epilepticus in susceptible patients. Oral rather than IV treatment is usually more appropriate, and the drugs of choice are valproate, lamotrigine, clonazepam, clobazam, and topiramate. Barbiturates, carbamazepine, gabapentin, tiagabine, and vigabatrin can worsen the episode.

8.4.4 **Myoclonic status epilepticus in coma**

Myoclonic status epilepticus in coma is the term used to describe the relatively common sequel of prolonged cerebral anoxia resulting from cardiorespiratory arrest (typically after a myocardial infarction or cardiac surgery). The patient in this situation is deeply comatose and with spontaneous and stimulus-sensitive myoclonus evident. To what extent this is really an 'epileptic' state, or is it simply a sign of severely damaged brain is arguable. The patients generally have periodic complexes on the EEG. The mortality rates are very high, and survivors may be left in a persistent vegetative state, or with severe neurological deficit or Lance–Adams type action myoclonus. Whether antiepileptic treatment influences the course of this condition is quite unclear. Some authorities recommend aggressive antiepileptic therapy and others none at all. Others recommend anti-status therapy for a 24hr period, often with high-dose barbiturate, but at this stage in the absence of any improvement, the antiepileptic therapy should then be withdrawn.

8.4.5 **Epilepsia Partialis Continua**

Epilepsia partialis continua (EPC) is a term used to describe what is approximately equivalent to focal motor status epilepticus. Spontaneous regular or irregular clonic twitching occurs, confined to one part of the body, and continuing for prolonged periods (often months or years). Consciousness is not impaired. There are many causes (Table 8.6) and the treatment should be largely directed at the underlying cause. For immunological conditions, therapy with steroids, high-dose IV immunoglobulin (IgG) or plasma exchange may be needed. The seizures can remit spontaneously in acute cases, although in well-established cases, EPC is very resistant to antiepileptic therapy. It is

Table 8.6 Some causes of epilepsia partialis continua (EPC)	
Immunological cerebral disorders	Rasmussen's encephalitis, SLE, other collagen diseases, celiac disease, auto-immune limbic encephalitis, paraneoplastic disease, granuloma
Structural cerebral disorders	Stroke, tumour, bacterial infection, HIV, viral encephalitis, Whipple disease, anoxic brain damage, cortical dysplasia
Mitochondrial disease	MELAS, MERFF, Alpers disease
Metabolic disease	Acute metabolic disturbance including non-ketotic hyperglycaemia
Other medical	Systemic infections, drugs, toxins, poisonings

HIV = human immunodeficiency virus; MELAS = mitochondrial myopathy encephalopathy lactic acidosis and stroke-like episodes; MERFF = myoclonus epilepsy with ragged-red fibres syndrome; SLE = systemic lupus erythematosus.

usual to prescribe oral antiepileptic drugs at least to prevent secondary generalization, even if the EPC itself is not controlled. The long-term outcome depends on the underlying cause, but in many cases the clonic movements continue in spite of medical therapy.

References

Aminoff MJ and Simon RP (1980). Status epilepticus. Causes, clinical features and consequences in 98 patients. *The American Journal of Medicine*, **69**, 657–66.

Brown JK and Hussain IH (1991). Status epilepticus. I: Pathogenesis. *Developmental Medicine and Child Neurology*, **33**, 3–17.

Cockerell OC, Rothwell J, Thompson PD, Marsden CD, and Shorvon SD (1996). Clinical and physiological features of epilepsia partialis continua. Cases ascertained in the UK. *Brain*, **119**(Pt 2), 393–407.

DeLorenzo RJ, Garnett LK, Towne AR, Waterhouse EJ, Boggs JG, Morton L, Choudhry MA, Barnes T, Ko D (1999). Comparison of status epilepticus with prolonged seizure episodes lasting from 10 to 29 minutes. *Epilepsia*, **40**, 164–9.

Leppik IE, Derivan AT, Homan RW, Walker J, Ramsay RE, and Patrick B (1983). Double-blind study of lorazepam and diazepam in status epilepticus. *JAMA*, **249**, 1452–4.

Lothman EW, Bertram EH, Bekenstein JW, and Perlin JB (1989). Self-sustaining limbic status epilepticus induced by 'continuous' hippocampal stimulation: electrographic and behavioral characteristics. *Epilepsy Research*, **3**, 107–19.

Meldrum BS and Brierley JB (1973). Prolonged epileptic seizures in primates. Ischemic cell change and its relation to ictal physiological events. *Archives of Neurology*, **28**, 10–17.

Meldrum BS and Horton RW (1973). Physiology of status epilepticus in primates. *Archives of Neurology*, **28**, 1–9.

Meldrum BS, Vigouroux RA, and Brierley JB (1973). Systemic factors and epileptic brain damage. Prolonged seizures in paralyzed, artificially ventilated baboons. *Archives of Neurology*, **29**, 82–7.

Scott RC, Besag FM, and Neville BG (1999). Buccal midazolam and rectal diazepam for treatment of prolonged seizures in childhood and adolescence: a randomised trial [see comments]. *Lancet*, **353**, 623–6.

Shaner DM, McCurdy SA, Herring MO, and Gabor AJ (1988). Treatment of status epilepticus: a prospective comparison of diazepam and phenytoin versus phenobarbital and optional phenytoin. *Neurology*, **38**, 202–7.

Shorvon SD (1994). *Status epilepticus in adults and children: its clinical features and treatment*. Cambridge University Press, Cambridge.

Shorvon SD (2000). *Handbook of epilepsy treatment*. Blackwell Science Ltd., Oxford.

Shorvon SD, Trinka E, and Walker MC (2007). Proceedings of the First London Colloquium on Status Epilepticus—University College London, April 12–15, 2007. *Epilepsia*, **48**, (S8), 1–109.

Simon RP (1985). Physiologic consequences of status epilepticus. *Epilepsia*, **26**(Suppl 1), S58–66.

Treiman DM, Meyers PD, Walton NY, Collins JF, Colling C, Rowan AJ, Handforth A, Faught E, Calabrese VP, Uthman BM, Ramsay RE, Mamdani MB (1998). A comparison of four treatments for generalized convulsive status epilepticus. Veterans Affairs Status Epilepticus Cooperative Study Group. *The New England Journal of Medicine*, **339**, 792–8.

Walker MC (2001). Diagnosis and treatment of nonconvulsive status epilepticus. *CNS Drugs*, **15**, 931–9.

Williamson PD, Spencer DD, Spencer SS, Novelly RA, and Mattson RH (1985). Complex partial status epilepticus: a depth-electrode study. *Annals of Neurology*, **18**, 647–54.

Chapter 9

Social and psychosocial aspects of epilepsy

Key points

- The psychosocial consequences of epilepsy and the permanent state of 'being epileptic' are often more problematic than the seizures themselves.
- Many psychosocial effects are dependent on societal, cultural, or personal factors and are amenable to improvement by counselling, psychotherapy, or support.
- The large Clinical Standards Advisory Group (CSAG) survey showed the extent to which different areas of concern were related to age and the severity of the epilepsy. In adults, common issues of concern are the driving ban, work, social life, psychological factors, impairment of memory, and loss of confidence. In children, common issues were school and education, psychological factors, social life, sports, the need to take tablets, sleep, supervision, play, and difficulties with learning.
- The lack of predictability of seizures is a major cause of loss of self-confidence and self-esteem, and undermines the confidence of people with epilepsy.
- The tendency for 'overprotection' and 'overdependency' should be avoided.
- Issues that commonly arise in a clinical setting relate to: death, friendships and relationships, reproductive issues, parenting, safety, employment, leisure, accidental injury, and schooling.
- Information provision, counselling, and psychotherapy can be very helpful in resolving these issues.
- The treating physician has a duty to convey the driving regulations to the patient where relevant.

Epilepsy is a condition in which the social and psychosocial secondary handicaps are sometime more problematic to the patient than the medical condition itself. 'Being epileptic' is a permanent state, whereas the seizures themselves may occur only occasionally and be very brief. The social and psychological effects of the condition are heavily influenced by cultural, societal, or personal factors, and many are amendable to improvement by counselling, psychotherapy, or support.

9.1 **The social and psychological impact of epilepsy**

This is a very large topic, and it is not possible in the space available to deal comprehensively with all aspects. What follows is a brief summary of just some of the non-medical aspects encountered in medical practice. It is also of course an absolute imperative to recognize that individuals have different needs, and thus to avoid generalizations; and a survey such as this will be inadequate to define specific aspects in any individual. Some common themes are outlined below, but the complexity of the interaction of an individual's epilepsy, personal qualities, environment, and upbringing defy simple analysis.

The problems caused by epilepsy differ at different stages of the condition, and also vary according to age and to the severity of the condition. A large population-based survey was carried out in Britain in 1999 to identify those areas in which the condition had its greatest impact, and the main impacts (and the proportion of patients reporting impacts) are summarized in Tables 9.1–9.3. The results were subdivided by age group and seizure severity (measured using the *National Hospital Seizure Severity Scale*). As can be seen, epilepsy had impacts in many areas of life, although these were much less amongst those with mild epilepsy. Not surprisingly, the areas of impact differed greatly at different ages.

Table 9.1 The CSAG survey—adult patients with mild seizures	
Area	Percentage of patients reporting a major impact in this area
Patients aged 17–65yrs with mild seizures[a]	
Driving ban	48
Work	36
Social life	19
Psychological	18
Loss of confidence	8
None	11

Table 9.1 (Contd)

Area	Percentage of patients reporting a major impact in this area
Patients aged >65yrs with mild seizures[b]	
Driving ban	32
Psychological	19
Work	14
Bad memory	9
None	19

CSAG = Clinical Standards Advisory Group.

Table shows the most commonly reported impacts.

Patients' seizures were divided into mild or severe on the basis of frequency and score on National Hospital Seizure Severity Scale; Derived from Moran et al. (1999).

[a] A total of 568 patients returned a questionnaire; impacts reported = 1,140.

[b] A total of 127 patients returned a questionnaire; impacts reported = 191.

Table 9.2 CSAG survey—adult patients with severe seizures

Area	Percentage of patients reporting a major impact in this area
Patients aged 17–65yrs with severe seizures[a]	
Work	51
Psychological	35
Social life	32
Driving ban	28
Supervision	10
Independence	9
Patients aged >65yrs with severe seizures[b]	
Driving ban	39
Psychological	29
Seizures	21
Work	21
Social life	14
Loss of self-confidence	11
Mobility	11
Supervision	11

CSAG = Clinical Standards Advisory Group.

Table shows the most commonly reported impacts.

Patients' seizures were divided into mild or severe on the basis of frequency and score on National Hospital Seizure Severity Scale; Derived from Moran et al. (1999).

[a] A total of 347 patients returned the questionnaire; impacts reported = 842.

[b] A total of 28 patients returned a questionnaire; impacts reported = 57.

Table 9.3 CSAG survey—patients under the age of 17yrs	
Area	Percentage of patients reporting a major impact in this area
Patients aged <17yrs with mild seizures[a]	
School life/education	36
Psychological	27
Social life	24
Sports	18
Need to take tablets	15
Sleep	9
Learning difficulties	9
None	9
Patients aged <17yrs with severe seizures[b]	
School life/education	33
Psychological	31
Social life	30
Sports	15
Supervision	11
Sleep	11
Play	7
Need to take tablets	7

CSAG = Clinical Standards Advisory Group.
Table shows the commonest reported impacts.
Patients' seizures were divided into mild or severe on the basis of frequency and score on National Hospital Seizure Severity Scale; Derived from Moran et al. (1999).
[a] A total of 33 patients returned the questionnaire; impacts reported = 61.
[b] A total of 54 patients returned a questionnaire; impacts reported = 121.

9.1.1 The lack of predictability of seizures and the assessment of risk

The fact that seizures occur in an unpredictable manner is often their most detrimental feature. This undermines the feeling of security and can have a devastating effect on confidence and self-esteem. Of all the psychological consequences of epilepsy, this is probably the most significant, can result in social withdrawal, excessive restriction, and underachievement, and it is essential to recognize these problems and to offer assistance. The avoidance of the secondary handicap caused in this way can make a big difference to a person's life, and yet requires great strength of character. Dependency and 'learned helplessness' are mechanisms sometimes employed by people faced with these problems; such responses are generally maladaptive, and should be countered especially in children and young adults.

All individuals with epilepsy need to draw a balance between accepting risk and accepting limitations—and where this line is drawn has to be an individual decision. Families or friends often err on the side of caution ('overprotection'). The epilepsy should be kept in context as much as possible, and it is important that the sufferer does not let the epilepsy unduly take over or dictate life decisions. These considerations are important in many areas of life, including social relationships, leisure activities, and choice of employment. The epilepsy should be seen as a challenge to be overcome as much as a handicap.

A vital goal for a person with epilepsy is to take control of the emotional and personal aspects of their life. Counselling can be very helpful in this regard, by talking through issues that arise.

9.1.2 **Death in epilepsy**

The possibility of death due to epilepsy is an important issue, which should be discussed with most patients. The occurrence of epilepsy carries with it a slightly higher annual mortality rate than would be expected in the general population, and a slightly reduced life expectancy. Death can be due to epilepsy in a number of ways. The underlying cause of the epilepsy may be fatal, for instance, in the case of a tumour. Death can also occur in a seizure due to 'SUDEP' (sudden unexpected death in epilepsy), an accident during a seizure or in status epilepticus. SUDEP occurs in the aftermath of a tonic-clonic seizures and the mechanism of death seems likely to be usually post-ictal failure of respiratory drive or cardiac arrhythmia. SUDEP occurs most commonly in seizures occurring in sleep and if the person is unaccompanied at the time of the seizure. The excess risk of SUDEP is approximately 1 per thousand per year overall, but falls to zero if the epilepsy is in remission and rises to 1 in 100 per year in patients with severe and frequent tonic-clonic seizures. The risk can be reduced by improving seizure control, by avoiding seizure precipitants, by reducing the risk of a seizure whilst unaccompanied especially at night, and by the use of alarms.

9.1.3 **Friendships and relationships**

Studies have shown that in broad terms, people with epilepsy have fewer relationships, have fewer friends, and are often more isolated than their peers. This is in part due to prejudice, but personal factors are also important. Epilepsy can engender low self-esteem and social withdrawal. Fear of prejudice may result in a perception of greater prejudice than is actually present. This can lead to anxiety over the forming of relationships and consequential social isolation; a vicious circle thus can result. There is also a danger of overdependency in some relationships, and of a relationship predicated on illness and dependency. This is potentially maladaptive and should generally be avoided. Sexual activity should not generally be affected by a diagnosis of epilepsy, although libido can sometimes be affected by the presence of epilepsy and also by drug treatment.

9.1.4 **Specific issues relating to contraception, fertility, pregnancy and childbirth**

There are a number of important issues relating to reproduction that affect women with epilepsy. These are dealt with in Chapter 5.

9.1.5 **Parenting**

Striking the balance between protecting the vulnerable child and allowing full normal activity is extremely difficult for the parent. The balance often is perceived by outsiders to be too risk-adverse, and there is a general tendency for parents to be considered to 'overprotect' the child. Although such overprotection may lessen the risk of injury, and also the risk of psychological trauma from unpleasant external events, it carries serious disadvantages. The child may feel, or indeed become, isolated; may not develop social graces; and may become overdependent. Personality development can be retarded. The child may underachieve and experience low self-esteem. Striking a balance is obviously difficult, but it is important that this issue is not ignored.

9.1.6 **Safety at home**

Most home activities carry little risk. However, if the epilepsy is active, and particularly if loss of consciousness occurs without warning, there are particular risks. A significant number of individuals die each year from drowning in baths. Showers are thus generally preferred, and if a bath is taken, it should be shallow, the bathroom door should remain unlocked, and someone in the house should be informed. There are also risks when cooking, and the use of a microwave is generally preferable to a cooker. Cooking with pans of hot oil or hot water should be avoided. Guards for open fires, radiators, and cookers are advisable. In severe epilepsy, there may be heightened concern about whether the person should live alone, whether accommodation is suitable (stairs, etc.), and whether dependant children are in a vulnerable position if seizures occur.

9.1.7 **Employment**

Most occupations can be followed by people with active epilepsy, and it is important to emphasis this. Epilepsy is covered by the Disability Discrimination Act (2005) in Britain which legislates against discrimination against people with epilepsy when applying for any job. There are furthermore relatively few jobs barred by statutory provision, and these include piloting aircraft, driving public service vehicles (ambulance, taxi, train), working as a merchant seaman, or as a frontline member of the armed forces. Other jobs however will carry obvious risks, for instance, working at heights or with unprotected machinery or working as a surgeon or anaesthetist. Common sense should apply when considering any post.

There is an obligation to disclose the condition to employers only if this could affect the ability to do the job or affect safety at work. Failure to disclose epilepsy in such circumstances can be used as grounds for dismissal and furthermore can invalidate the employers' liability. However, if a seizure is likely to occur at work, even if the seizure would have no effect on the ability to carry out the duties of the post, it is in general terms usually better to disclose the diagnosis to an employer and to workmates.

When initially applying for a position, unless the epilepsy is likely to have a significant effect on an individual's ability to do the job, there is no obligation to disclose the condition unless specifically asked. However, it is generally best to mention the condition before accepting the job offer or at final interview. In doing so, it is important to put this in a realistic but favourable light. A supportive letter from the General Practitioner or hospital doctor will often help. In larger organizations, where there is an occupational health department, an assessment by this department can be carried out independently of line management.

The prejudice perceived by people with epilepsy when applying for jobs is sometimes greater than the actual prejudice. Ignorance of the facts about epilepsy, rather than prejudice, is often at the root of many negative attitudes. Furthermore, a failure to obtain a post will often depend on other factors—for instance, a person's attitude, personality, and confidence. It is essential at an interview for the person not to dwell overly on the negative aspects of the epilepsy.

9.1.8 **Leisure activities**

Most leisure activities can be undertaken and indeed are to be encouraged for the gain in confidence that might result, the enjoyment derived, and beneficial effects on friendships and personality development. In most circumstances, the social and psychological damage done by restricting a person's life probably outstrips the risks. Sensible precautions should be taken. Swimming, for instance, is perfectly possible, but preferably in the company of someone who could attend to the individual if a seizure occurs, and the pool lifeguard should be informed. Such activities as cycling, rock climbing, and horse riding should be allowed in most cases (depending on the nature of the seizures) but usually in the company of someone who knows about the epilepsy or in an organized group and with appropriate safety equipment.

9.1.9 **Accidental injury**

People with uncontrolled epilepsy with falls are at risk of head and facial injuries, and in severe cases, a protective helmet is advisable.

159

There is also an increased incidence of limb fractures and accidental dermatological and other injuries amongst persons with epilepsy. The injuries are more common in those with falls occurring in a tonic phase of a seizure and in those in whom the fall occurs without warning. Injury is, not surprising, commoner in those with severe epilepsy. Sensible precautions should be taken where possible.

9.1.10 **Schooling**

Most children with epilepsy attend normal schools. Only the minority who have additional learning difficulties or who have very severe epilepsy require special education.

However, many children with epilepsy underachieve at school. There are a number of reasons for this, some biological and some social. The epilepsy itself may be responsible, by causing drowsiness or cognitive impairment, or in the case of absence seizures, by constantly interrupting the flow of consciousness. Antiepileptic drugs can impair cognitive functions although this impairment should be a relatively slight, in most patients, with skilful drug therapy. Low expectations can play an important part, and the expectation of failure or poor performance can become self-fulfilling. 'Overprotection' of children with epilepsy is another common problem. It is important that neither teachers nor parents restrict activities of a child unnecessarily. Teachers should be aware of possible teasing and bullying, and take a firm line to counter this. If it is likely that a child will have a seizure at school, then often it is worth educating the class about seizures and epilepsy.

9.2 **Counselling and information provision**

It is imperative that relevant information is freely available to all patients with epilepsy. In newly diagnosed epilepsy, information will be needed on many medical and personal aspects. The medical topics listed in Box 9.1 should be covered in all patients. A particular issue concerns the need for good compliance with medication. Advice needs also to be given about legal aspects such as those that relate to the driving regulations. The personal advice needed will depend on individual circumstances and on the stage or severity of the epilepsy.

In newly diagnosed epilepsy, adjustment to a diagnosis of epilepsy can be a major issue. This is usually a gradual process which can be difficult. A feeling of loss (of good health, of previous life circumstances) is often a prominent feature. The belief that the individual

> **Box 9.1 Medical topics for information provision and counselling for all patients with epilepsy**
>
> - Nature of epilepsy
> - First aid management of seizures
> - Avoidance of precipitating factors, including alcohol and sleep deprivation
> - Purpose of medication, and the likely duration of treatment
> - Nature of common adverse effects of medication
> - Need to take medication regularly
> - Risks of seizures (including sudden unexpected death in epilepsy [SUDEP]), and advice regarding common hazards
> - Interaction with other drugs

has lost control and the resulting feeling of powerlessness can lead to social withdrawal, loss of self-esteem, and to dependency. Anxiety or depression can occur. In some cases, denial leading to poor compliance with medication is a problem, and can further disrupt the process of adjustment. These issues are particularly prominent in adolescence.

In chronic epilepsy, counselling on a broader range of personal topics is often needed. Issues of safety and risk are usually more pressing and decisions need to be taken about where to draw the line in relation to risk. This is, as mentioned earlier, a personal decision and counselling can be very helpful by articulating the issues and defining the choices. Commonly, advice is needed on such aspects as education, employment, benefits and rights, domestic arrangements, travel, leisure, sexual activity, contraception, emotional aspects, relationships, issues relating to child-rearing and pregnancy, death, co-morbidity, and psychiatric conditions.

Information needs to be accessible and special efforts can be required to meet the needs of disadvantaged groups or those with special requirements—for instance, those from ethnic groups where the first language is not that of the country in which they reside, people with learning disabilities and those with poor literacy skills. Time is needed to provide the full range of information required which is often not available in a doctors' clinic setting. Specialist epilepsy nurses or counsellors trained in epilepsy can provide invaluable service in this regard. Written information is available from many sources (e.g. clinical information, web-based information, and publications from the voluntary sector) and is an important adjunct to personal counselling.

9.3 **Driving**

Driving is one of the few areas in which, in many countries, legislation exists specifically in relation to epilepsy. The rules differ from country to country and indeed in the United States, from state to state. In general, persons with active epilepsy are prohibited from driving until a minimum period of seizure freedom has occurred (this period in usually 1–2yrs although in some US states it is as little as 3 months). Driving is prohibited in active epilepsy because of the obvious risk of having a seizure at the wheel of a motor vehicle. There are many surveys showing that people with a history of epilepsy have higher rates of accidents. There is also a higher rate of unlawful driving, and an epileptic fit has also been shown to be the second most common cause of a driver fatality categorised as 'collapse at the wheel' (myocardial infarction is the commonest cause).

Here, the UK regulations will be outlined, which are similar (but not the same) to those in many countries in Europe. In the United Kingdom, it is the role of a government agency—the Driving and Vehicle Licensing Agency (DVLA)—to issue driving licenses. The individual licence holder is under an obligation to notify the DVLA if an epileptic seizure occurs. The DVLA has the power to withhold or withdraw licensing if a seizure occurs, and the rules differ for different types of vehicle:

9.3.1 **Rules for a Group 1 Licence (a normal driving licence for car and motorcycles)**

A person who has had an epileptic attack while awake must refrain from driving for 12 months from the date of the attack before a driving licence may be issued. A person who has had an attack while asleep must also refrain from driving for 12 months from the date of the attack, unless attacks have occurred only whilst asleep over the preceding 3yr period during which time no awake attacks have occurred.

In addition, the person must comply with the advised treatment and check-ups for epilepsy, and the driving of a vehicle by such a person should not be likely to cause danger to the public.

9.3.2 **Rules for a Group 2 License (which cover most lorries, buses, and taxis)**

The rules are much stricter. The following three conditions must all be met during the period of 10yrs immediately preceding the date when the licence is granted: the applicant should have been free from any epileptic attack (asleep or awake); must have not required or taken any medication to treat epilepsy; and should not otherwise be a source of danger while driving.

9.3.3 **Other points**

A person having a solitary seizure must normally satisfy the afore-mentioned regulations.

A person with a structural intracranial lesion who has an increased risk of seizures will not be able to drive vehicles of this group until the risk of a seizure has fallen to no greater than 2% per annum.

The aforementioned rules apply to 'epileptic' seizures. For the purposes of the legislation, a provoked or acute symptomatic seizure is not considered necessarily to be 'epileptic' by the DVLA and may be dealt with on an individual basis, provided there is no previous seizure history. The decision to prohibit driving in this situation will be influenced by such aspects as whether the provoking stimulus carries any risk of recurrence or whether the stimulus had been successfully or appropriately treated or was unlikely to occur at the wheel. For example, the following seizures are usually considered provoked: eclamptic seizures; reflex anoxic seizures; an immediate seizure at the time of a head injury; a seizure in the first week following a head injury, which is not associated with any damage on computer tomography (CT) scanning or with post-traumatic amnesia of longer than 30min; a seizure at the time of a stroke/transient ischemic attack (TIA) or within the ensuing 24hrs; and a seizure occurring during intracranial surgery or in the ensuing 24hrs. Seizures associated with alcohol or drug misuse, sleep deprivation, or a structural abnormality are not considered as 'provoked' for licensing purposes.

9.3.4 **The role of the doctor in relation to the driving regulations**

In Britain, the doctor is generally not involved in decisions about whether or not licensing should be permitted—this role is devolved to the DVLA. This is an excellent way of avoiding the conflict that can arise by mixing medical with licensing issues. Furthermore, medical notes are confidential and cannot be divulged to the DVLA without the written consent of the patient.

The main duty of the doctor is to make it clear to a driving licence holder that the condition may affect their safety as a driver, and that the driver has a *legal duty* to inform the DVLA about the condition.

In the extreme case, where a patient refuses to inform the DVLA (for instance, by refusing to accept the diagnosis or the effect of the condition on the ability to drive), the breaking of rules of confidentiality can be considered. The doctor should advise the patient not to drive, and if this advice is disputed, a second opinion is often useful to obtain. If the patient continues to drive when not fit to do so, the doctor should make every reasonable effort to dissuade driving. The advice should be recorded in writing and copied in writing to the patient. If the patient continues to drive despite the aforementioned measures, the doctor then has a duty to disclose relevant medical information, in confidence, to the DVLA. Before giving information to the DVLA, the doctor should inform the patient of the decision to do so. Once the DVLA has been informed, the doctor should also write to the patient to say that a disclosure has been made.

References and further reading

Attarian H, Vahle V, Carter J, Hykes E, and Gilliam F (2003). Relationship between depression and intractability of seizures. *Epilepsy & behaviour*, **4**, 298–301.

Baker GA, Jacoby A, Buck D, Gilliam FG, Harden CL, Hermann B, Kanner AM, Caplan R, Plioplys S, Salpekar J, Dunn D, Austin J, Jones J (1997). Quality of life of people with epilepsy: a European study. *Epilepsia*, **38**, 353–62.

Barry JJ, Ettinger AB, and Friel P (2008). Consensus statement: the evaluation and treatment of people with epilepsy and affective disorders. *Epilepsy & behaviour*, **13**(Suppl 1),S1–29.

Bell GS, Nashef L, and Kendall S (2002). Information recalled by women taking anti-epileptic drugs for epilepsy: a questionnaire study. *Epilepsy Research*, **52**, 139–46.

Clinical Standards Advisory Group (2000). *Services for people with epilepsy*. Department of Health, London.

Drivers Medical Group, DVLA (2007). *At a glance guide to the current medical standards of fitness to drive*. DVLA, Swansea.

Jacoby A, Baker GA, Steen N, Potts P, Chadwick DW. (1996). The clinical course of epilepsy and its psychosocial correlates: findings from a U.K. Community study. *Epilepsia*, **37**, 148–61.

Jones JE, Hermann BP, Barry JJ, Gilliam FG, Kanner AM, and Meador KJ (2003). Rates and risk factors for suicide, suicidal ideation, and suicide attempts in chronic epilepsy. *Epilepsy & behaviour*, **4**(Suppl 3), S31–8.

Kobau R, Gilliam F, and Thurman DJ (2006). Prevalence of self-reported epilepsy or seizure disorder and its associations with self-reported depression and anxiety: results from the 2004 HealthStyles Survey. *Epilepsia*, **47**, 1915–21.

Gilliam F (2003). The impact of epilepsy on subjective health status. *Current Neurology and Neuroscience Reports*, **3**, 357–62.

Gilliam F, Kuzniecky R, Faught E, Black L, Carpenter G, Schrodt R (1997). Patient-validated content of epilepsy-specific quality-of-life measurement. *Epilepsia*, **38**, 233–6.

Gilliam F, Carter J, and Vahle V (2004). Tolerability of antiseizure medications: implications for health outcomes. *Neurology*, **63**(Suppl 4), S9–12.

Gilliam FG and Santos JM (2006). Adverse psychiatric effects of antiepileptic drugs. *Epilepsy Research*, **68**, 67–9.

Jacoby A (1992). Epilepsy and the quality of everyday life. Findings from a study of people with well-controlled epilepsy. *Social Science & Medicine*, **34**, 657–66.

Moran N, Poole K, and Bell GJ et al. (2000). NHS services for epilepsy from the patient's perspective: a survey of primary, secondary and tertiary care access throughout the UK. *Seizure*, **9**, 559–65.

Moran NF, Poole K, and Bell GJ et al. (2004). Epilepsy in the United Kingdom: seizure frequency and severity, anti-epileptic drug utilization and impact on life in 1652 people with epilepsy. *Seizure*, **13**, 425–33.

O'Donoghue MF, Duncan JS, and Sander JW (1996). The National Hospital Seizure Severity Scale: a further development of the Chalfont Seizure Severity Scale. *Epilepsia*, **37**, 563–71.

O'Donoghue MF, Duncan JS, and Sander JW (1998). The subjective handicap of epilepsy. A new approach to measuring treatment outcome. *Brain*, 121, 317–43.

Panayiotopoulos CP (2004). *The epilepsies: seizures, syndromes and management*. Bladon Medical Publishing, London.

Poole K, Moran N, and Bell GJ et al. (2000). Patients' perspectives on services for epilepsy: a survey of patient satisfaction, preferences and information provision in 2394 people with epilepsy. *Seizure*, **9**, 551–8.

Wallace SJ and Farrell K (eds). (2004). *Epilepsy in children*. Arnold, London.

Index